THIS BOOK BELONGS TO:

CONTACT INFORMATION

NAME:	
ADDRESS:	
PHONE:	

START / END DATES

___ / ___ / ___   TO   ___ / ___ / ___

DEDICATION

This Coffee Tasting Journal log is dedicated to all the Coffee Lovers out there who love tasting different coffees and document their findings in the process.

You are my inspiration for producing books and I'm honored to be a part of keeping all of your coffee notes and records organized.

This journal notebook will help you record your details about your coffee tasting adventures.

Thoughtfully put together with these sections to record in detail: Coffee Name & Brand, Date & Place Tasted, Price Beverage, Country/ Region Origin & Company, Testing Rating, Brew Method, Recommended, & Notes.

HOW TO USE THIS BOOK

The purpose of this book is to keep all of your Coffee Tasting notes all in one place. It will help keep you organized.

This Coffee Tasting Journal will allow you to accurately document every detail about tasting different coffees. It's a great way to chart your course through recording your coffee adventures.

Here are examples of the prompts for you to fill in and write about your experience in this book:

1. **Coffee Name/ Brand** - Log the Name & Brand of your Coffee.

2. **Date & Place Tasted** - Record the Date & Place you tasted.

3. **Price** - Write the cost of your purchase.

4. **Beverage** - Which style of coffee.

5. **Country/ Region Origin, Company**

6. **Testing Rating** - Rate Appearance, Aroma, Flavor, Sweet, Acidic, Spicy, Citrus, Chocolate, Caramel, Bitter & Savory by coloring the rating scale from .5 to 5

7. **Brew Method** - Check boxes to check the brewing type: Drip, Espresso, Press, Pour Over, Siphon or Other.

8. **Recommended To** - Do you recommend this bean blend.

9. **Notes** - Blank lined, great for writing your personal favorites or favorite cup, your coffee tasting adventures, your coffee recipe idea, etc.

COFFEE NAME _____ DATE _____

BEVERAGE _____

PLACE TASTED _____ PRICE _____

COUNTRY / REGION _____

COMPANY _____

TESTING RATING

	0.5	1	1.5	2	2.5	3	3.5	4	4.5	5
APPEARANCE										
AROMA										
FLAVOR										

	0.5	1	1.5	2	2.5	3	3.5	4	4.5	5
SWEET										
ACIDIC										
SPICY										
CITRUS										
CHOCOLATE										
CARAMEL										
BITTER										
SAVORY										

BREW METHOD

DRIP ☐   ESPRESSO ☐   PRESS ☐

POUR-OVER ☐   SIPHON ☐   OTHER _____

NOTES _____

RECOMMEND TO _____

COFFEE NAME _____   DATE _____

BEVERAGE _____

PLACE TASTED _____   PRICE _____

COUNTRY / REGION _____

COMPANY _____

TESTING RATING

	0.5	1	1.5	2	2.5	3	3.5	4	4.5	5
APPEARANCE										
AROMA										
FLAVOR										

	0.5	1	1.5	2	2.5	3	3.5	4	4.5	5
SWEET										
ACIDIC										
SPICY										
CITRUS										
CHOCOLATE										
CARAMEL										
BITTER										
SAVORY										

BREW METHOD

DRIP ☐   ESPRESSO ☐   PRESS ☐

POUR-OVER ☐   SIPHON ☐   OTHER _____

NOTES _____

_____
_____
_____
_____
_____
_____
_____
_____
_____

RECOMMEND TO _____

_____
_____
_____
_____
_____
_____
_____
_____
_____

COFFEE NAME _____   DATE _____

BEVERAGE _____

PLACE TASTED _____   PRICE _____

COUNTRY / REGION _____

COMPANY _____

TESTING RATING

	0.5	1	1.5	2	2.5	3	3.5	4	4.5	5
APPEARANCE										
AROMA										
FLAVOR										

	0.5	1	1.5	2	2.5	3	3.5	4	4.5	5
SWEET										
ACIDIC										
SPICY										
CITRUS										
CHOCOLATE										
CARAMEL										
BITTER										
SAVORY										

BREW METHOD

DRIP ☐   ESPRESSO ☐   PRESS ☐

POUR-OVER ☐   SIPHON ☐   OTHER _____

NOTES _____

_____
_____
_____
_____
_____
_____
_____
_____
_____
_____

RECOMMEND TO _____

_____
_____
_____
_____
_____
_____
_____
_____
_____
_____

COFFEE NAME _____ DATE _____

BEVERAGE _____

PLACE TASTED _____ PRICE _____

COUNTRY / REGION _____

COMPANY _____

TESTING RATING

```
              0.5 1 1.5 2 2.5 3 3.5 4 4.5 5
APPEARANCE   [                              ]
AROMA        [                              ]
FLAVOR       [                              ]
```

```
            0.5 1 1.5 2 2.5 3 3.5 4 4.5 5
SWEET      [                              ]
ACIDIC     [                              ]
SPICY      [                              ]
CITRUS     [                              ]
CHOCOLATE  [                              ]
CARAMEL    [                              ]
BITTER     [                              ]
SAVORY     [                              ]
```

BREW METHOD

DRIP ☐ ESPRESSO ☐ PRESS ☐

POUR-OVER ☐ SIPHON ☐ OTHER _____

NOTES _____

RECOMMEND TO _____

COFFEE NAME _____ DATE _____

BEVERAGE _____

PLACE TASTED _____ PRICE _____

COUNTRY / REGION _____

COMPANY _____

TESTING RATING

	0.5	1	1.5	2	2.5	3	3.5	4	4.5	5
APPEARANCE										
AROMA										
FLAVOR										

	0.5	1	1.5	2	2.5	3	3.5	4	4.5	5
SWEET										
ACIDIC										
SPICY										
CITRUS										
CHOCOLATE										
CARAMEL										
BITTER										
SAVORY										

BREW METHOD

DRIP ☐   ESPRESSO ☐   PRESS ☐

POUR-OVER ☐   SIPHON ☐   OTHER _____

NOTES _____

_____
_____
_____
_____
_____
_____
_____
_____
_____
_____

RECOMMEND TO _____

_____
_____
_____
_____
_____
_____
_____
_____
_____
_____

COFFEE NAME _____ **DATE** _____

BEVERAGE _____

PLACE TASTED _____   **PRICE** _____

COUNTRY / REGION _____

COMPANY _____

TESTING RATING

```
              0.5  1  1.5  2  2.5  3  3.5  4  4.5  5
APPEARANCE   [                                      ]
AROMA        [                                      ]
FLAVOR       [                                      ]
```

```
              0.5  1  1.5  2  2.5  3  3.5  4  4.5  5
SWEET        [                                      ]
ACIDIC       [                                      ]
SPICY        [                                      ]
CITRUS       [                                      ]
CHOCOLATE    [                                      ]
CARAMEL      [                                      ]
BITTER       [                                      ]
SAVORY       [                                      ]
```

BREW METHOD

DRIP ☐   ESPRESSO ☐   PRESS ☐

POUR-OVER ☐   SIPHON ☐   OTHER _____

NOTES _____
_____
_____
_____
_____
_____
_____
_____
_____

RECOMMEND TO _____
_____
_____
_____
_____
_____
_____
_____
_____

COFFEE NAME _____ DATE _____

BEVERAGE _____

PLACE TASTED _____ PRICE _____

COUNTRY / REGION _____

COMPANY _____

TESTING RATING

	0.5	1	1.5	2	2.5	3	3.5	4	4.5	5
APPEARANCE										
AROMA										
FLAVOR										

BREW METHOD

DRIP ☐   ESPRESSO ☐   PRESS ☐

POUR-OVER ☐   SIPHON ☐   OTHER _____

	0.5	1	1.5	2	2.5	3	3.5	4	4.5	5
SWEET										
ACIDIC										
SPICY										
CITRUS										
CHOCOLATE										
CARAMEL										
BITTER										
SAVORY										

NOTES _____

_____

_____

_____

_____

_____

_____

_____

_____

_____

RECOMMEND TO _____

_____

_____

_____

_____

_____

_____

_____

_____

_____

COFFEE NAME _____ DATE _____

BEVERAGE _____

PLACE TASTED _____ PRICE _____

COUNTRY / REGION _____

COMPANY _____

TESTING RATING

	0.5	1	1.5	2	2.5	3	3.5	4	4.5	5
APPEARANCE										
AROMA										
FLAVOR										

	0.5	1	1.5	2	2.5	3	3.5	4	4.5	5
SWEET										
ACIDIC										
SPICY										
CITRUS										
CHOCOLATE										
CARAMEL										
BITTER										
SAVORY										

BREW METHOD

DRIP ☐ ESPRESSO ☐ PRESS ☐

POUR-OVER ☐ SIPHON ☐ OTHER _____

NOTES _____

_____
_____
_____
_____
_____
_____
_____
_____
_____
_____

RECOMMEND TO _____

_____
_____
_____
_____
_____
_____
_____
_____
_____
_____

COFFEE NAME _____ **DATE** _____

BEVERAGE _____

PLACE TASTED _____ **PRICE** _____

COUNTRY / REGION _____

COMPANY _____

TESTING RATING

	0.5	1	1.5	2	2.5	3	3.5	4	4.5	5
APPEARANCE										
AROMA										
FLAVOR										

	0.5	1	1.5	2	2.5	3	3.5	4	4.5	5
SWEET										
ACIDIC										
SPICY										
CITRUS										
CHOCOLATE										
CARAMEL										
BITTER										
SAVORY										

BREW METHOD

DRIP ☐   ESPRESSO ☐   PRESS ☐

POUR-OVER ☐   SIPHON ☐   OTHER _____

NOTES _____
_____
_____
_____
_____
_____
_____
_____
_____
_____

RECOMMEND TO _____
_____
_____
_____
_____
_____
_____
_____
_____
_____

COFFEE NAME _____ **DATE** _____

BEVERAGE _____

PLACE TASTED _____ **PRICE** _____

COUNTRY / REGION _____

COMPANY _____

TESTING RATING

```
              0.5  1  1.5  2  2.5  3  3.5  4  4.5  5
APPEARANCE   [                                      ]
AROMA        [                                      ]
FLAVOR       [                                      ]
```

```
           0.5  1  1.5  2  2.5  3  3.5  4  4.5  5
SWEET     [                                      ]
ACIDIC    [                                      ]
SPICY     [                                      ]
CITRUS    [                                      ]
CHOCOLATE [                                      ]
CARAMEL   [                                      ]
BITTER    [                                      ]
SAVORY    [                                      ]
```

BREW METHOD

DRIP ☐   ESPRESSO ☐   PRESS ☐

POUR-OVER ☐   SIPHON ☐   OTHER _____

NOTES _____

_____
_____
_____
_____
_____
_____
_____
_____

RECOMMEND TO _____

_____
_____
_____
_____
_____
_____
_____
_____

COFFEE NAME _____   DATE _____

BEVERAGE _____

PLACE TASTED _____   PRICE _____

COUNTRY / REGION _____

COMPANY _____

TESTING RATING

	0.5	1	1.5	2	2.5	3	3.5	4	4.5	5
APPEARANCE										
AROMA										
FLAVOR										

	0.5	1	1.5	2	2.5	3	3.5	4	4.5	5
SWEET										
ACIDIC										
SPICY										
CITRUS										
CHOCOLATE										
CARAMEL										
BITTER										
SAVORY										

BREW METHOD

DRIP ☐   ESPRESSO ☐   PRESS ☐

POUR-OVER ☐   SIPHON ☐   OTHER _____

NOTES _____

_____
_____
_____
_____
_____
_____
_____
_____
_____
_____

RECOMMEND TO _____

_____
_____
_____
_____
_____
_____
_____
_____
_____
_____

COFFEE NAME _____ DATE _____

BEVERAGE _____

PLACE TASTED _____ PRICE _____

COUNTRY / REGION _____

COMPANY _____

TESTING RATING

```
              0.5  1  1.5  2  2.5  3  3.5  4  4.5  5
APPEARANCE  [                                      ]
AROMA       [                                      ]
FLAVOR      [                                      ]
```

```
           0.5  1  1.5  2  2.5  3  3.5  4  4.5  5
SWEET     [                                      ]
ACIDIC    [                                      ]
SPICY     [                                      ]
CITRUS    [                                      ]
CHOCOLATE [                                      ]
CARAMEL   [                                      ]
BITTER    [                                      ]
SAVORY    [                                      ]
```

BREW METHOD

DRIP ☐   ESPRESSO ☐   PRESS ☐

POUR-OVER ☐   SIPHON ☐   OTHER _____

NOTES _____

_____
_____
_____
_____
_____
_____
_____
_____
_____

RECOMMEND TO _____

_____
_____
_____
_____
_____
_____
_____
_____
_____

COFFEE NAME _____ DATE _____

BEVERAGE _____

PLACE TASTED _____   PRICE _____

COUNTRY / REGION _____

COMPANY _____

TESTING RATING

	0.5	1	1.5	2	2.5	3	3.5	4	4.5	5
APPEARANCE										
AROMA										
FLAVOR										

	0.5	1	1.5	2	2.5	3	3.5	4	4.5	5
SWEET										
ACIDIC										
SPICY										
CITRUS										
CHOCOLATE										
CARAMEL										
BITTER										
SAVORY										

BREW METHOD

DRIP ☐   ESPRESSO ☐   PRESS ☐

POUR-OVER ☐   SIPHON ☐   OTHER _____

NOTES _____

RECOMMEND TO _____

COFFEE NAME _____ DATE _____

BEVERAGE _____

PLACE TASTED _____ PRICE _____

COUNTRY / REGION _____

COMPANY _____

TESTING RATING

	0.5 1 1.5 2 2.5 3 3.5 4 4.5 5
APPEARANCE	☐☐☐☐☐☐☐☐☐☐
AROMA	☐☐☐☐☐☐☐☐☐☐
FLAVOR	☐☐☐☐☐☐☐☐☐☐

	0.5 1 1.5 2 2.5 3 3.5 4 4.5 5
SWEET	☐☐☐☐☐☐☐☐☐☐
ACIDIC	☐☐☐☐☐☐☐☐☐☐
SPICY	☐☐☐☐☐☐☐☐☐☐
CITRUS	☐☐☐☐☐☐☐☐☐☐
CHOCOLATE	☐☐☐☐☐☐☐☐☐☐
CARAMEL	☐☐☐☐☐☐☐☐☐☐
BITTER	☐☐☐☐☐☐☐☐☐☐
SAVORY	☐☐☐☐☐☐☐☐☐☐

BREW METHOD

DRIP ☐   ESPRESSO ☐   PRESS ☐

POUR-OVER ☐   SIPHON ☐   OTHER _____

NOTES _____

_____
_____
_____
_____
_____
_____
_____
_____
_____

RECOMMEND TO _____

_____
_____
_____
_____
_____
_____
_____
_____
_____

COFFEE NAME _____ **DATE** _____

BEVERAGE _____

PLACE TASTED _____ **PRICE** _____

COUNTRY / REGION _____

COMPANY _____

TESTING RATING

	0.5	1	1.5	2	2.5	3	3.5	4	4.5	5
APPEARANCE										
AROMA										
FLAVOR										

	0.5	1	1.5	2	2.5	3	3.5	4	4.5	5
SWEET										
ACIDIC										
SPICY										
CITRUS										
CHOCOLATE										
CARAMEL										
BITTER										
SAVORY										

BREW METHOD

DRIP ☐ ESPRESSO ☐ PRESS ☐

POUR-OVER ☐ SIPHON ☐ OTHER _____

NOTES _____

_____
_____
_____
_____
_____
_____
_____
_____
_____
_____

RECOMMEND TO _____

_____
_____
_____
_____
_____
_____
_____
_____
_____
_____

COFFEE NAME _____ DATE _____

BEVERAGE _____

PLACE TASTED _____ PRICE _____

COUNTRY / REGION _____

COMPANY _____

TESTING RATING

```
              0.5  1  1.5  2  2.5  3  3.5  4  4.5  5
APPEARANCE  [                                        ]
AROMA       [                                        ]
FLAVOR      [                                        ]
```

```
          0.5  1  1.5  2  2.5  3  3.5  4  4.5  5
SWEET     [                                        ]
ACIDIC    [                                        ]
SPICY     [                                        ]
CITRUS    [                                        ]
CHOCOLATE [                                        ]
CARAMEL   [                                        ]
BITTER    [                                        ]
SAVORY    [                                        ]
```

BREW METHOD

DRIP ☐   ESPRESSO ☐   PRESS ☐

POUR-OVER ☐   SIPHON ☐   OTHER _____

NOTES _____

RECOMMEND TO _____

COFFEE NAME _____ DATE _____

BEVERAGE _____

PLACE TASTED _____ PRICE _____

COUNTRY / REGION _____

COMPANY _____

TESTING RATING

	0.5	1	1.5	2	2.5	3	3.5	4	4.5	5
APPEARANCE										
AROMA										
FLAVOR										

	0.5	1	1.5	2	2.5	3	3.5	4	4.5	5
SWEET										
ACIDIC										
SPICY										
CITRUS										
CHOCOLATE										
CARAMEL										
BITTER										
SAVORY										

BREW METHOD

DRIP ☐   ESPRESSO ☐   PRESS ☐

POUR-OVER ☐   SIPHON ☐   OTHER _____

NOTES _____

RECOMMEND TO _____

COFFEE NAME _____ DATE _____

BEVERAGE _____

PLACE TASTED _____ PRICE _____

COUNTRY / REGION _____

COMPANY _____

TESTING RATING

```
              0.5  1  1.5  2  2.5  3  3.5  4  4.5  5
APPEARANCE   [                                      ]
AROMA        [                                      ]
FLAVOR       [                                      ]
```

```
              0.5  1  1.5  2  2.5  3  3.5  4  4.5  5
SWEET        [                                      ]
ACIDIC       [                                      ]
SPICY        [                                      ]
CITRUS       [                                      ]
CHOCOLATE    [                                      ]
CARAMEL      [                                      ]
BITTER       [                                      ]
SAVORY       [                                      ]
```

BREW METHOD

DRIP ☐   ESPRESSO ☐   PRESS ☐

POUR-OVER ☐   SIPHON ☐   OTHER _____

NOTES _____

_____
_____
_____
_____
_____
_____
_____
_____

RECOMMEND TO _____

_____
_____
_____
_____
_____
_____
_____
_____

COFFEE NAME _____ DATE _____

BEVERAGE _____

PLACE TASTED _____   PRICE _____

COUNTRY / REGION _____

COMPANY _____

TESTING RATING

	0.5	1	1.5	2	2.5	3	3.5	4	4.5	5
APPEARANCE										
AROMA										
FLAVOR										

	0.5	1	1.5	2	2.5	3	3.5	4	4.5	5
SWEET										
ACIDIC										
SPICY										
CITRUS										
CHOCOLATE										
CARAMEL										
BITTER										
SAVORY										

BREW METHOD

DRIP ☐   ESPRESSO ☐   PRESS ☐

POUR-OVER ☐   SIPHON ☐   OTHER _____

NOTES _____
_____
_____
_____
_____
_____
_____
_____
_____
_____
_____

RECOMMEND TO _____
_____
_____
_____
_____
_____
_____
_____
_____
_____
_____

COFFEE NAME _____   DATE _____

BEVERAGE _____

PLACE TASTED _____   PRICE _____

COUNTRY / REGION _____

COMPANY _____

TESTING RATING

	0.5	1	1.5	2	2.5	3	3.5	4	4.5	5
APPEARANCE										
AROMA										
FLAVOR										

	0.5	1	1.5	2	2.5	3	3.5	4	4.5	5
SWEET										
ACIDIC										
SPICY										
CITRUS										
CHOCOLATE										
CARAMEL										
BITTER										
SAVORY										

BREW METHOD

DRIP ☐   ESPRESSO ☐   PRESS ☐

POUR-OVER ☐   SIPHON ☐   OTHER _____

NOTES _____

_____
_____
_____
_____
_____
_____
_____
_____
_____
_____

RECOMMEND TO _____

_____
_____
_____
_____
_____
_____
_____
_____
_____
_____

COFFEE NAME _____ DATE _____

BEVERAGE _____

PLACE TASTED _____ PRICE _____

COUNTRY / REGION _____

COMPANY _____

TESTING RATING

```
                 0.5  1  1.5  2  2.5  3  3.5  4  4.5  5
APPEARANCE   [                                          ]
AROMA        [                                          ]
FLAVOR       [                                          ]
```

```
                 0.5  1  1.5  2  2.5  3  3.5  4  4.5  5
SWEET        [                                          ]
ACIDIC       [                                          ]
SPICY        [                                          ]
CITRUS       [                                          ]
CHOCOLATE    [                                          ]
CARAMEL      [                                          ]
BITTER       [                                          ]
SAVORY       [                                          ]
```

BREW METHOD

DRIP ☐   ESPRESSO ☐   PRESS ☐

POUR-OVER ☐   SIPHON ☐   OTHER _____

NOTES _____

_____
_____
_____
_____
_____
_____
_____
_____
_____
_____
_____

RECOMMEND TO _____

_____
_____
_____
_____
_____
_____
_____
_____
_____
_____
_____

COFFEE NAME _____ **DATE** _____

BEVERAGE _____

PLACE TASTED _____ **PRICE** _____

COUNTRY / REGION _____

COMPANY _____

TESTING RATING

	0.5	1	1.5	2	2.5	3	3.5	4	4.5	5
APPEARANCE										
AROMA										
FLAVOR										

	0.5	1	1.5	2	2.5	3	3.5	4	4.5	5
SWEET										
ACIDIC										
SPICY										
CITRUS										
CHOCOLATE										
CARAMEL										
BITTER										
SAVORY										

BREW METHOD

DRIP ☐   ESPRESSO ☐   PRESS ☐

POUR-OVER ☐   SIPHON ☐   OTHER _____

NOTES _____

_____
_____
_____
_____
_____
_____
_____
_____
_____
_____

RECOMMEND TO _____

_____
_____
_____
_____
_____
_____
_____
_____
_____
_____

COFFEE NAME _____ **DATE** _____

BEVERAGE _____

PLACE TASTED _____ **PRICE** _____

COUNTRY / REGION _____

COMPANY _____

TESTING RATING

	0.5	1	1.5	2	2.5	3	3.5	4	4.5	5
APPEARANCE										
AROMA										
FLAVOR										

	0.5	1	1.5	2	2.5	3	3.5	4	4.5	5
SWEET										
ACIDIC										
SPICY										
CITRUS										
CHOCOLATE										
CARAMEL										
BITTER										
SAVORY										

BREW METHOD

DRIP ☐   ESPRESSO ☐   PRESS ☐

POUR-OVER ☐   SIPHON ☐   OTHER _____

NOTES _____

_____
_____
_____
_____
_____
_____
_____
_____
_____
_____

RECOMMEND TO _____

_____
_____
_____
_____
_____
_____
_____
_____
_____
_____

COFFEE NAME _____   DATE _____

BEVERAGE _____

PLACE TASTED _____   PRICE _____

COUNTRY / REGION _____

COMPANY _____

TESTING RATING

```
                0.5  1  1.5  2  2.5  3  3.5  4  4.5  5
APPEARANCE  [                                         ]
AROMA       [                                         ]
FLAVOR      [                                         ]
```

```
                0.5  1  1.5  2  2.5  3  3.5  4  4.5  5
SWEET       [                                         ]
ACIDIC      [                                         ]
SPICY       [                                         ]
CITRUS      [                                         ]
CHOCOLATE   [                                         ]
CARAMEL     [                                         ]
BITTER      [                                         ]
SAVORY      [                                         ]
```

BREW METHOD

DRIP ☐   ESPRESSO ☐   PRESS ☐

POUR-OVER ☐   SIPHON ☐   OTHER _____

NOTES _____

RECOMMEND TO _____

COFFEE NAME _____ DATE _____

BEVERAGE _____

PLACE TASTED _____   PRICE _____

COUNTRY / REGION _____

COMPANY _____

TESTING RATING

	0.5	1	1.5	2	2.5	3	3.5	4	4.5	5
APPEARANCE										
AROMA										
FLAVOR										

BREW METHOD

DRIP ☐   ESPRESSO ☐   PRESS ☐

POUR-OVER ☐   SIPHON ☐   OTHER _____

	0.5	1	1.5	2	2.5	3	3.5	4	4.5	5
SWEET										
ACIDIC										
SPICY										
CITRUS										
CHOCOLATE										
CARAMEL										
BITTER										
SAVORY										

NOTES _____

_____
_____
_____
_____
_____
_____
_____
_____
_____
_____
_____

RECOMMEND TO _____

_____
_____
_____
_____
_____
_____
_____
_____
_____
_____
_____

COFFEE NAME _____   DATE _____

BEVERAGE _____

PLACE TASTED _____   PRICE _____

COUNTRY / REGION _____

COMPANY _____

TESTING RATING

```
              0.5  1  1.5  2  2.5  3  3.5  4  4.5  5
APPEARANCE  [                                        ]
AROMA       [                                        ]
FLAVOR      [                                        ]
```

```
           0.5  1  1.5  2  2.5  3  3.5  4  4.5  5
SWEET     [                                        ]
ACIDIC    [                                        ]
SPICY     [                                        ]
CITRUS    [                                        ]
CHOCOLATE [                                        ]
CARAMEL   [                                        ]
BITTER    [                                        ]
SAVORY    [                                        ]
```

BREW METHOD

DRIP ☐   ESPRESSO ☐   PRESS ☐

POUR-OVER ☐   SIPHON ☐   OTHER _____

NOTES _____

RECOMMEND TO _____

COFFEE NAME _____   **DATE** _____

BEVERAGE _____

PLACE TASTED _____   **PRICE** _____

COUNTRY / REGION _____

COMPANY _____

TESTING RATING

	0.5	1	1.5	2	2.5	3	3.5	4	4.5	5
APPEARANCE										
AROMA										
FLAVOR										

	0.5	1	1.5	2	2.5	3	3.5	4	4.5	5
SWEET										
ACIDIC										
SPICY										
CITRUS										
CHOCOLATE										
CARAMEL										
BITTER										
SAVORY										

BREW METHOD

DRIP ☐   ESPRESSO ☐   PRESS ☐

POUR-OVER ☐   SIPHON ☐   OTHER _____

NOTES _____
_____
_____
_____
_____
_____
_____
_____
_____
_____

RECOMMEND TO _____
_____
_____
_____
_____
_____
_____
_____
_____
_____

COFFEE NAME _____ **DATE** _____

BEVERAGE _____

PLACE TASTED _____ **PRICE** _____

COUNTRY / REGION _____

COMPANY _____

TESTING RATING

```
              0.5  1  1.5  2  2.5  3  3.5  4  4.5  5
APPEARANCE   [                                      ]
AROMA        [                                      ]
FLAVOR       [                                      ]
```

```
              0.5  1  1.5  2  2.5  3  3.5  4  4.5  5
SWEET        [                                      ]
ACIDIC       [                                      ]
SPICY        [                                      ]
CITRUS       [                                      ]
CHOCOLATE    [                                      ]
CARAMEL      [                                      ]
BITTER       [                                      ]
SAVORY       [                                      ]
```

BREW METHOD

DRIP ☐   ESPRESSO ☐   PRESS ☐

POUR-OVER ☐   SIPHON ☐   OTHER _____

NOTES _____
_____
_____
_____
_____
_____
_____
_____
_____
_____

RECOMMEND TO _____
_____
_____
_____
_____
_____
_____
_____
_____
_____

COFFEE NAME _____ **DATE** _____

BEVERAGE _____

PLACE TASTED _____ **PRICE** _____

COUNTRY / REGION _____

COMPANY _____

TESTING RATING

	0.5	1	1.5	2	2.5	3	3.5	4	4.5	5
APPEARANCE										
AROMA										
FLAVOR										

	0.5	1	1.5	2	2.5	3	3.5	4	4.5	5
SWEET										
ACIDIC										
SPICY										
CITRUS										
CHOCOLATE										
CARAMEL										
BITTER										
SAVORY										

BREW METHOD

DRIP ☐   ESPRESSO ☐   PRESS ☐

POUR-OVER ☐   SIPHON ☐   OTHER _____

NOTES _____

_____

_____

_____

_____

_____

_____

_____

_____

_____

RECOMMEND TO _____

_____

_____

_____

_____

_____

_____

_____

_____

_____

COFFEE NAME _____ DATE _____

BEVERAGE _____

PLACE TASTED _____ PRICE _____

COUNTRY / REGION _____

COMPANY _____

TESTING RATING

	0.5	1	1.5	2	2.5	3	3.5	4	4.5	5
APPEARANCE										
AROMA										
FLAVOR										

	0.5	1	1.5	2	2.5	3	3.5	4	4.5	5
SWEET										
ACIDIC										
SPICY										
CITRUS										
CHOCOLATE										
CARAMEL										
BITTER										
SAVORY										

BREW METHOD

DRIP ☐   ESPRESSO ☐   PRESS ☐

POUR-OVER ☐   SIPHON ☐   OTHER _____

NOTES _____

_____
_____
_____
_____
_____
_____
_____
_____
_____
_____

RECOMMEND TO _____

_____
_____
_____
_____
_____
_____
_____
_____
_____
_____

COFFEE NAME _____ **DATE** _____

BEVERAGE _____

PLACE TASTED _____ **PRICE** _____

COUNTRY / REGION _____

COMPANY _____

TESTING RATING

```
              0.5  1  1.5  2  2.5  3  3.5  4  4.5  5
APPEARANCE  [                                       ]
AROMA       [                                       ]
FLAVOR      [                                       ]
```

BREW METHOD

DRIP ☐   ESPRESSO ☐   PRESS ☐
POUR-OVER ☐   SIPHON ☐   OTHER _____

```
           0.5  1  1.5  2  2.5  3  3.5  4  4.5  5
SWEET     [                                       ]
ACIDIC    [                                       ]
SPICY     [                                       ]
CITRUS    [                                       ]
CHOCOLATE [                                       ]
CARAMEL   [                                       ]
BITTER    [                                       ]
SAVORY    [                                       ]
```

NOTES _____

RECOMMEND TO _____

COFFEE NAME _____ DATE _____

BEVERAGE _____

PLACE TASTED _____ PRICE _____

COUNTRY / REGION _____

COMPANY _____

TESTING RATING

```
              0.5  1  1.5  2  2.5  3  3.5  4  4.5  5
APPEARANCE   [                                      ]
AROMA        [                                      ]
FLAVOR       [                                      ]
```

```
             0.5  1  1.5  2  2.5  3  3.5  4  4.5  5
SWEET       [                                      ]
ACIDIC      [                                      ]
SPICY       [                                      ]
CITRUS      [                                      ]
CHOCOLATE   [                                      ]
CARAMEL     [                                      ]
BITTER      [                                      ]
SAVORY      [                                      ]
```

BREW METHOD

DRIP ☐   ESPRESSO ☐   PRESS ☐

POUR-OVER ☐   SIPHON ☐   OTHER _____

NOTES _____

_____
_____
_____
_____
_____
_____
_____
_____
_____

RECOMMEND TO _____

_____
_____
_____
_____
_____
_____
_____
_____
_____

COFFEE NAME _____ DATE _____

BEVERAGE _____

PLACE TASTED _____   PRICE _____

COUNTRY / REGION _____

COMPANY _____

TESTING RATING

```
              0.5  1  1.5  2  2.5  3  3.5  4  4.5  5
APPEARANCE   [                                      ]
AROMA        [                                      ]
FLAVOR       [                                      ]
```

```
              0.5  1  1.5  2  2.5  3  3.5  4  4.5  5
SWEET        [                                      ]
ACIDIC       [                                      ]
SPICY        [                                      ]
CITRUS       [                                      ]
CHOCOLATE    [                                      ]
CARAMEL      [                                      ]
BITTER       [                                      ]
SAVORY       [                                      ]
```

BREW METHOD

DRIP ☐   ESPRESSO ☐   PRESS ☐

POUR-OVER ☐   SIPHON ☐   OTHER _____

NOTES _____

_____
_____
_____
_____
_____
_____
_____
_____
_____
_____

RECOMMEND TO _____

_____
_____
_____
_____
_____
_____
_____
_____
_____
_____

COFFEE NAME _____ DATE _____

BEVERAGE _____

PLACE TASTED _____ PRICE _____

COUNTRY / REGION _____

COMPANY _____

TESTING RATING

```
              0.5  1  1.5  2  2.5  3  3.5  4  4.5  5
APPEARANCE  [                                        ]
AROMA       [                                        ]
FLAVOR      [                                        ]
```

```
           0.5  1  1.5  2  2.5  3  3.5  4  4.5  5
SWEET     [                                        ]
ACIDIC    [                                        ]
SPICY     [                                        ]
CITRUS    [                                        ]
CHOCOLATE [                                        ]
CARAMEL   [                                        ]
BITTER    [                                        ]
SAVORY    [                                        ]
```

BREW METHOD

DRIP ☐   ESPRESSO ☐   PRESS ☐

POUR-OVER ☐   SIPHON ☐   OTHER _____

NOTES _____

_____
_____
_____
_____
_____
_____
_____
_____
_____
_____

RECOMMEND TO _____

_____
_____
_____
_____
_____
_____
_____
_____
_____
_____

COFFEE NAME _____   DATE _____

BEVERAGE _____

PLACE TASTED _____   PRICE _____

COUNTRY / REGION _____

COMPANY _____

TESTING RATING

```
              0.5  1  1.5  2  2.5  3  3.5  4  4.5  5
APPEARANCE  [                                        ]
AROMA       [                                        ]
FLAVOR      [                                        ]
```

```
              0.5  1  1.5  2  2.5  3  3.5  4  4.5  5
SWEET       [                                        ]
ACIDIC      [                                        ]
SPICY       [                                        ]
CITRUS      [                                        ]
CHOCOLATE   [                                        ]
CARAMEL     [                                        ]
BITTER      [                                        ]
SAVORY      [                                        ]
```

BREW METHOD

DRIP ☐   ESPRESSO ☐   PRESS ☐

POUR-OVER ☐   SIPHON ☐   OTHER _____

NOTES _____

_____
_____
_____
_____
_____
_____
_____
_____
_____
_____

RECOMMEND TO _____

_____
_____
_____
_____
_____
_____
_____
_____
_____
_____

COFFEE NAME _____ DATE _____

BEVERAGE _____

PLACE TASTED _____ PRICE _____

COUNTRY / REGION _____

COMPANY _____

TESTING RATING

	0.5	1	1.5	2	2.5	3	3.5	4	4.5	5
APPEARANCE										
AROMA										
FLAVOR										

	0.5	1	1.5	2	2.5	3	3.5	4	4.5	5
SWEET										
ACIDIC										
SPICY										
CITRUS										
CHOCOLATE										
CARAMEL										
BITTER										
SAVORY										

BREW METHOD

DRIP ☐   ESPRESSO ☐   PRESS ☐

POUR-OVER ☐   SIPHON ☐   OTHER _____

NOTES _____

_____
_____
_____
_____
_____
_____
_____
_____
_____

RECOMMEND TO _____

_____
_____
_____
_____
_____
_____
_____
_____
_____

COFFEE NAME _____ DATE _____

BEVERAGE _____

PLACE TASTED _____ PRICE _____

COUNTRY / REGION _____

COMPANY _____

TESTING RATING

	0.5	1	1.5	2	2.5	3	3.5	4	4.5	5
APPEARANCE										
AROMA										
FLAVOR										

BREW METHOD

DRIP ☐   ESPRESSO ☐   PRESS ☐

POUR-OVER ☐   SIPHON ☐   OTHER _____

	0.5	1	1.5	2	2.5	3	3.5	4	4.5	5
SWEET										
ACIDIC										
SPICY										
CITRUS										
CHOCOLATE										
CARAMEL										
BITTER										
SAVORY										

NOTES _____

_____
_____
_____
_____
_____
_____
_____
_____
_____
_____
_____
_____

RECOMMEND TO _____

_____
_____
_____
_____
_____
_____
_____
_____
_____
_____
_____
_____

COFFEE NAME _____ DATE _____

BEVERAGE _____

PLACE TASTED _____ PRICE _____

COUNTRY / REGION _____

COMPANY _____

TESTING RATING

```
              0.5  1  1.5  2  2.5  3  3.5  4  4.5  5
APPEARANCE  [                                        ]
AROMA       [                                        ]
FLAVOR      [                                        ]
```

```
            0.5  1  1.5  2  2.5  3  3.5  4  4.5  5
SWEET     [                                        ]
ACIDIC    [                                        ]
SPICY     [                                        ]
CITRUS    [                                        ]
CHOCOLATE [                                        ]
CARAMEL   [                                        ]
BITTER    [                                        ]
SAVORY    [                                        ]
```

BREW METHOD

DRIP ☐   ESPRESSO ☐   PRESS ☐

POUR-OVER ☐   SIPHON ☐   OTHER _____

NOTES _____

_____
_____
_____
_____
_____
_____
_____
_____
_____
_____

RECOMMEND TO _____

_____
_____
_____
_____
_____
_____
_____
_____
_____
_____

COFFEE NAME _____ DATE _____

BEVERAGE _____

PLACE TASTED _____ PRICE _____

COUNTRY / REGION _____

COMPANY _____

TESTING RATING

	0.5	1	1.5	2	2.5	3	3.5	4	4.5	5
APPEARANCE										
AROMA										
FLAVOR										

	0.5	1	1.5	2	2.5	3	3.5	4	4.5	5
SWEET										
ACIDIC										
SPICY										
CITRUS										
CHOCOLATE										
CARAMEL										
BITTER										
SAVORY										

BREW METHOD

DRIP ☐   ESPRESSO ☐   PRESS ☐

POUR-OVER ☐   SIPHON ☐   OTHER _____

NOTES _____
_____
_____
_____
_____
_____
_____
_____
_____
_____
_____

RECOMMEND TO _____
_____
_____
_____
_____
_____
_____
_____
_____
_____
_____

COFFEE NAME _____ **DATE** _____

BEVERAGE _____

PLACE TASTED _____ **PRICE** _____

COUNTRY / REGION _____

COMPANY _____

TESTING RATING

	0.5	1	1.5	2	2.5	3	3.5	4	4.5	5
APPEARANCE										
AROMA										
FLAVOR										

	0.5	1	1.5	2	2.5	3	3.5	4	4.5	5
SWEET										
ACIDIC										
SPICY										
CITRUS										
CHOCOLATE										
CARAMEL										
BITTER										
SAVORY										

BREW METHOD

DRIP ☐   ESPRESSO ☐   PRESS ☐

POUR-OVER ☐   SIPHON ☐   OTHER _____

NOTES _____

_____
_____
_____
_____
_____
_____
_____
_____
_____

RECOMMEND TO _____

_____
_____
_____
_____
_____
_____
_____
_____
_____

COFFEE NAME _____ DATE _____

BEVERAGE _____

PLACE TASTED _____ PRICE _____

COUNTRY / REGION _____

COMPANY _____

TESTING RATING

	0.5	1	1.5	2	2.5	3	3.5	4	4.5	5
APPEARANCE										
AROMA										
FLAVOR										

	0.5	1	1.5	2	2.5	3	3.5	4	4.5	5
SWEET										
ACIDIC										
SPICY										
CITRUS										
CHOCOLATE										
CARAMEL										
BITTER										
SAVORY										

BREW METHOD

DRIP ☐ ESPRESSO ☐ PRESS ☐

POUR-OVER ☐ SIPHON ☐ OTHER _____

NOTES _____

RECOMMEND TO _____

COFFEE NAME _____ DATE _____

BEVERAGE _____

PLACE TASTED _____ PRICE _____

COUNTRY / REGION _____

COMPANY _____

TESTING RATING

```
                0.5  1  1.5  2  2.5  3  3.5  4  4.5  5
APPEARANCE     [                                      ]
AROMA          [                                      ]
FLAVOR         [                                      ]
```

```
                0.5  1  1.5  2  2.5  3  3.5  4  4.5  5
SWEET          [                                      ]
ACIDIC         [                                      ]
SPICY          [                                      ]
CITRUS         [                                      ]
CHOCOLATE      [                                      ]
CARAMEL        [                                      ]
BITTER         [                                      ]
SAVORY         [                                      ]
```

BREW METHOD

DRIP ☐   ESPRESSO ☐   PRESS ☐

POUR-OVER ☐   SIPHON ☐   OTHER _____

NOTES _____

_____
_____
_____
_____
_____
_____
_____
_____
_____

RECOMMEND TO _____

_____
_____
_____
_____
_____
_____
_____
_____
_____

COFFEE NAME _____ **DATE** _____

BEVERAGE _____

PLACE TASTED _____ **PRICE** _____

COUNTRY / REGION _____

COMPANY _____

TESTING RATING

	0.5	1	1.5	2	2.5	3	3.5	4	4.5	5
APPEARANCE										
AROMA										
FLAVOR										

	0.5	1	1.5	2	2.5	3	3.5	4	4.5	5
SWEET										
ACIDIC										
SPICY										
CITRUS										
CHOCOLATE										
CARAMEL										
BITTER										
SAVORY										

BREW METHOD

DRIP ☐   ESPRESSO ☐   PRESS ☐

POUR-OVER ☐   SIPHON ☐   OTHER _____

NOTES _____

_____

_____

_____

_____

_____

_____

_____

_____

RECOMMEND TO _____

_____

_____

_____

_____

_____

_____

_____

_____

COFFEE NAME _____ DATE _____

BEVERAGE _____

PLACE TASTED _____ PRICE _____

COUNTRY / REGION _____

COMPANY _____

TESTING RATING

	0.5	1	1.5	2	2.5	3	3.5	4	4.5	5
APPEARANCE										
AROMA										
FLAVOR										

	0.5	1	1.5	2	2.5	3	3.5	4	4.5	5
SWEET										
ACIDIC										
SPICY										
CITRUS										
CHOCOLATE										
CARAMEL										
BITTER										
SAVORY										

BREW METHOD

DRIP ☐   ESPRESSO ☐   PRESS ☐

POUR-OVER ☐   SIPHON ☐   OTHER _____

NOTES _____

_____
_____
_____
_____
_____
_____
_____
_____
_____

RECOMMEND TO _____

_____
_____
_____
_____
_____
_____
_____
_____
_____

COFFEE NAME _____ DATE _____

BEVERAGE _____

PLACE TASTED _____   PRICE _____

COUNTRY / REGION _____

COMPANY _____

TESTING RATING

	0.5	1	1.5	2	2.5	3	3.5	4	4.5	5
APPEARANCE										
AROMA										
FLAVOR										

	0.5	1	1.5	2	2.5	3	3.5	4	4.5	5
SWEET										
ACIDIC										
SPICY										
CITRUS										
CHOCOLATE										
CARAMEL										
BITTER										
SAVORY										

BREW METHOD

DRIP ☐   ESPRESSO ☐   PRESS ☐

POUR-OVER ☐   SIPHON ☐   OTHER _____

NOTES _____
_____
_____
_____
_____
_____
_____
_____
_____
_____

RECOMMEND TO _____
_____
_____
_____
_____
_____
_____
_____
_____
_____

COFFEE NAME _____ DATE _____

BEVERAGE _____

PLACE TASTED _____ PRICE _____

COUNTRY / REGION _____

COMPANY _____

TESTING RATING

	0.5 1 1.5 2 2.5 3 3.5 4 4.5 5		0.5 1 1.5 2 2.5 3 3.5 4 4.5 5
APPEARANCE	▭▭▭▭▭▭▭▭▭▭	SWEET	▭▭▭▭▭▭▭▭▭▭
AROMA	▭▭▭▭▭▭▭▭▭▭	ACIDIC	▭▭▭▭▭▭▭▭▭▭
FLAVOR	▭▭▭▭▭▭▭▭▭▭	SPICY	▭▭▭▭▭▭▭▭▭▭
		CITRUS	▭▭▭▭▭▭▭▭▭▭
		CHOCOLATE	▭▭▭▭▭▭▭▭▭▭
		CARAMEL	▭▭▭▭▭▭▭▭▭▭
		BITTER	▭▭▭▭▭▭▭▭▭▭
		SAVORY	▭▭▭▭▭▭▭▭▭▭

BREW METHOD

DRIP ☐ ESPRESSO ☐ PRESS ☐

POUR-OVER ☐ SIPHON ☐ OTHER _____

NOTES _____

_____
_____
_____
_____
_____
_____
_____
_____
_____

RECOMMEND TO _____

_____
_____
_____
_____
_____
_____
_____
_____
_____

COFFEE NAME _____ DATE _____

BEVERAGE _____

PLACE TASTED _____ PRICE _____

COUNTRY / REGION _____

COMPANY _____

TESTING RATING

	0.5	1	1.5	2	2.5	3	3.5	4	4.5	5
APPEARANCE										
AROMA										
FLAVOR										

	0.5	1	1.5	2	2.5	3	3.5	4	4.5	5
SWEET										
ACIDIC										
SPICY										
CITRUS										
CHOCOLATE										
CARAMEL										
BITTER										
SAVORY										

BREW METHOD

DRIP ☐ ESPRESSO ☐ PRESS ☐

POUR-OVER ☐ SIPHON ☐ OTHER _____

NOTES _____

_____
_____
_____
_____
_____
_____
_____
_____
_____
_____
_____
_____

RECOMMEND TO _____

_____
_____
_____
_____
_____
_____
_____
_____
_____
_____
_____
_____

COFFEE NAME _____ DATE _____

BEVERAGE _____

PLACE TASTED _____ PRICE _____

COUNTRY / REGION _____

COMPANY _____

TESTING RATING

```
                0.5  1  1.5  2  2.5  3  3.5  4  4.5  5
APPEARANCE  [                                         ]
AROMA       [                                         ]
FLAVOR      [                                         ]
```

BREW METHOD

DRIP ☐   ESPRESSO ☐   PRESS ☐

POUR-OVER ☐   SIPHON ☐   OTHER _____

```
            0.5  1  1.5  2  2.5  3  3.5  4  4.5  5
SWEET     [                                         ]
ACIDIC    [                                         ]
SPICY     [                                         ]
CITRUS    [                                         ]
CHOCOLATE [                                         ]
CARAMEL   [                                         ]
BITTER    [                                         ]
SAVORY    [                                         ]
```

NOTES _____

_____
_____
_____
_____
_____
_____
_____
_____

RECOMMEND TO _____

_____
_____
_____
_____
_____
_____
_____
_____

COFFEE NAME _____ DATE _____

BEVERAGE _____

PLACE TASTED _____ PRICE _____

COUNTRY / REGION _____

COMPANY _____

TESTING RATING

	0.5	1	1.5	2	2.5	3	3.5	4	4.5	5
APPEARANCE										
AROMA										
FLAVOR										

	0.5	1	1.5	2	2.5	3	3.5	4	4.5	5
SWEET										
ACIDIC										
SPICY										
CITRUS										
CHOCOLATE										
CARAMEL										
BITTER										
SAVORY										

BREW METHOD

DRIP ☐   ESPRESSO ☐   PRESS ☐

POUR-OVER ☐   SIPHON ☐   OTHER _____

NOTES _____

_____
_____
_____
_____
_____
_____
_____
_____
_____
_____
_____

RECOMMEND TO _____

_____
_____
_____
_____
_____
_____
_____
_____
_____
_____
_____

COFFEE NAME _____   **DATE** _____

BEVERAGE _____

PLACE TASTED _____   **PRICE** _____

COUNTRY / REGION _____

COMPANY _____

TESTING RATING

	0.5	1	1.5	2	2.5	3	3.5	4	4.5	5
APPEARANCE										
AROMA										
FLAVOR										

	0.5	1	1.5	2	2.5	3	3.5	4	4.5	5
SWEET										
ACIDIC										
SPICY										
CITRUS										
CHOCOLATE										
CARAMEL										
BITTER										
SAVORY										

BREW METHOD

DRIP ☐   ESPRESSO ☐   PRESS ☐

POUR-OVER ☐   SIPHON ☐   OTHER _____

NOTES _____

_____
_____
_____
_____
_____
_____
_____
_____
_____
_____

RECOMMEND TO _____

_____
_____
_____
_____
_____
_____
_____
_____
_____
_____

COFFEE NAME _____ DATE _____

BEVERAGE _____

PLACE TASTED _____ PRICE _____

COUNTRY / REGION _____

COMPANY _____

TESTING RATING

```
              0.5  1  1.5  2  2.5  3  3.5  4  4.5  5
APPEARANCE  [                                        ]
AROMA       [                                        ]
FLAVOR      [                                        ]
```

```
              0.5  1  1.5  2  2.5  3  3.5  4  4.5  5
SWEET       [                                        ]
ACIDIC      [                                        ]
SPICY       [                                        ]
CITRUS      [                                        ]
CHOCOLATE   [                                        ]
CARAMEL     [                                        ]
BITTER      [                                        ]
SAVORY      [                                        ]
```

BREW METHOD

DRIP ☐   ESPRESSO ☐   PRESS ☐

POUR-OVER ☐   SIPHON ☐   OTHER _____

NOTES _____

RECOMMEND TO _____

COFFEE NAME _____ DATE _____

BEVERAGE _____

PLACE TASTED _____ PRICE _____

COUNTRY / REGION _____

COMPANY _____

TESTING RATING

```
              0.5  1  1.5  2  2.5  3  3.5  4  4.5  5
APPEARANCE  [                                        ]
AROMA       [                                        ]
FLAVOR      [                                        ]
```

```
              0.5  1  1.5  2  2.5  3  3.5  4  4.5  5
SWEET       [                                        ]
ACIDIC      [                                        ]
SPICY       [                                        ]
CITRUS      [                                        ]
CHOCOLATE   [                                        ]
CARAMEL     [                                        ]
BITTER      [                                        ]
SAVORY      [                                        ]
```

BREW METHOD

DRIP ☐   ESPRESSO ☐   PRESS ☐

POUR-OVER ☐   SIPHON ☐   OTHER _____

NOTES _____
_____
_____
_____
_____
_____
_____
_____
_____
_____

RECOMMEND TO _____
_____
_____
_____
_____
_____
_____
_____
_____
_____

COFFEE NAME _____ DATE _____

BEVERAGE _____

PLACE TASTED _____ PRICE _____

COUNTRY / REGION _____

COMPANY _____

TESTING RATING

	0.5 1 1.5 2 2.5 3 3.5 4 4.5 5
APPEARANCE	
AROMA	
FLAVOR	

	0.5 1 1.5 2 2.5 3 3.5 4 4.5 5
SWEET	
ACIDIC	
SPICY	
CITRUS	
CHOCOLATE	
CARAMEL	
BITTER	
SAVORY	

BREW METHOD

DRIP ☐   ESPRESSO ☐   PRESS ☐

POUR-OVER ☐   SIPHON ☐   OTHER _____

NOTES _____

RECOMMEND TO _____

COFFEE NAME _____   DATE _____

BEVERAGE _____

PLACE TASTED _____   PRICE _____

COUNTRY / REGION _____

COMPANY _____

TESTING RATING

	0.5	1	1.5	2	2.5	3	3.5	4	4.5	5
APPEARANCE										
AROMA										
FLAVOR										

	0.5	1	1.5	2	2.5	3	3.5	4	4.5	5
SWEET										
ACIDIC										
SPICY										
CITRUS										
CHOCOLATE										
CARAMEL										
BITTER										
SAVORY										

BREW METHOD

DRIP ☐   ESPRESSO ☐   PRESS ☐

POUR-OVER ☐   SIPHON ☐   OTHER _____

NOTES _____

_____
_____
_____
_____
_____
_____
_____
_____
_____
_____

RECOMMEND TO _____

_____
_____
_____
_____
_____
_____
_____
_____
_____
_____

COFFEE NAME _____ **DATE** _____

BEVERAGE _____

PLACE TASTED _____ **PRICE** _____

COUNTRY / REGION _____

COMPANY _____

TESTING RATING

	0.5	1	1.5	2	2.5	3	3.5	4	4.5	5
APPEARANCE										
AROMA										
FLAVOR										

	0.5	1	1.5	2	2.5	3	3.5	4	4.5	5
SWEET										
ACIDIC										
SPICY										
CITRUS										
CHOCOLATE										
CARAMEL										
BITTER										
SAVORY										

BREW METHOD

DRIP ☐   ESPRESSO ☐   PRESS ☐

POUR-OVER ☐   SIPHON ☐   OTHER _____

NOTES _____

_____
_____
_____
_____
_____
_____
_____
_____
_____

RECOMMEND TO _____

_____
_____
_____
_____
_____
_____
_____
_____
_____

COFFEE NAME _____ DATE _____

BEVERAGE _____

PLACE TASTED _____ PRICE _____

COUNTRY / REGION _____

COMPANY _____

TESTING RATING

```
              0.5  1  1.5  2  2.5  3  3.5  4  4.5  5
APPEARANCE  [                                        ]
AROMA       [                                        ]
FLAVOR      [                                        ]
```

BREW METHOD

DRIP ☐   ESPRESSO ☐   PRESS ☐

POUR-OVER ☐   SIPHON ☐   OTHER _____

```
            0.5  1  1.5  2  2.5  3  3.5  4  4.5  5
SWEET     [                                        ]
ACIDIC    [                                        ]
SPICY     [                                        ]
CITRUS    [                                        ]
CHOCOLATE [                                        ]
CARAMEL   [                                        ]
BITTER    [                                        ]
SAVORY    [                                        ]
```

NOTES _____

_____
_____
_____
_____
_____
_____
_____
_____
_____
_____

RECOMMEND TO _____

_____
_____
_____
_____
_____
_____
_____
_____
_____
_____

| COFFEE NAME | | DATE | |

BEVERAGE _____

PLACE TASTED _____ **PRICE** _____

COUNTRY / REGION _____

COMPANY _____

TESTING RATING

```
              0.5  1  1.5  2  2.5  3  3.5  4  4.5  5
APPEARANCE  [                                       ]
AROMA       [                                       ]
FLAVOR      [                                       ]
```

```
              0.5  1  1.5  2  2.5  3  3.5  4  4.5  5
SWEET      [                                       ]
ACIDIC     [                                       ]
SPICY      [                                       ]
CITRUS     [                                       ]
CHOCOLATE  [                                       ]
CARAMEL    [                                       ]
BITTER     [                                       ]
SAVORY     [                                       ]
```

BREW METHOD

DRIP ☐   ESPRESSO ☐   PRESS ☐

POUR-OVER ☐   SIPHON ☐   OTHER _____

NOTES _____

_____
_____
_____
_____
_____
_____
_____
_____
_____

RECOMMEND TO _____

_____
_____
_____
_____
_____
_____
_____
_____
_____

COFFEE NAME _____ DATE _____

BEVERAGE _____

PLACE TASTED _____ PRICE _____

COUNTRY / REGION _____

COMPANY _____

TESTING RATING

	0.5	1	1.5	2	2.5	3	3.5	4	4.5	5
APPEARANCE										
AROMA										
FLAVOR										

	0.5	1	1.5	2	2.5	3	3.5	4	4.5	5
SWEET										
ACIDIC										
SPICY										
CITRUS										
CHOCOLATE										
CARAMEL										
BITTER										
SAVORY										

BREW METHOD

DRIP ☐   ESPRESSO ☐   PRESS ☐

POUR-OVER ☐   SIPHON ☐   OTHER _____

NOTES _____

RECOMMEND TO _____

COFFEE NAME _____ DATE _____

BEVERAGE _____

PLACE TASTED _____ PRICE _____

COUNTRY / REGION _____

COMPANY _____

TESTING RATING

	0.5	1	1.5	2	2.5	3	3.5	4	4.5	5
APPEARANCE										
AROMA										
FLAVOR										

	0.5	1	1.5	2	2.5	3	3.5	4	4.5	5
SWEET										
ACIDIC										
SPICY										
CITRUS										
CHOCOLATE										
CARAMEL										
BITTER										
SAVORY										

BREW METHOD

DRIP ☐ ESPRESSO ☐ PRESS ☐

POUR-OVER ☐ SIPHON ☐ OTHER _____

NOTES _____
_____
_____
_____
_____
_____
_____
_____
_____
_____
_____
_____

RECOMMEND TO _____
_____
_____
_____
_____
_____
_____
_____
_____
_____
_____
_____
_____

COFFEE NAME _____   DATE _____

BEVERAGE _____

PLACE TASTED _____   PRICE _____

COUNTRY / REGION _____

COMPANY _____

TESTING RATING

```
               0.5  1  1.5  2  2.5  3  3.5  4  4.5  5
APPEARANCE    [                                      ]
AROMA         [                                      ]
FLAVOR        [                                      ]
```

```
               0.5  1  1.5  2  2.5  3  3.5  4  4.5  5
SWEET         [                                      ]
ACIDIC        [                                      ]
SPICY         [                                      ]
CITRUS        [                                      ]
CHOCOLATE     [                                      ]
CARAMEL       [                                      ]
BITTER        [                                      ]
SAVORY        [                                      ]
```

BREW METHOD

DRIP ☐   ESPRESSO ☐   PRESS ☐

POUR-OVER ☐   SIPHON ☐   OTHER _____

NOTES _____

_____
_____
_____
_____
_____
_____
_____
_____
_____

RECOMMEND TO _____

_____
_____
_____
_____
_____
_____
_____
_____
_____

COFFEE NAME _____ DATE _____

BEVERAGE _____

PLACE TASTED _____ PRICE _____

COUNTRY / REGION _____

COMPANY _____

TESTING RATING

	0.5	1	1.5	2	2.5	3	3.5	4	4.5	5
APPEARANCE										
AROMA										
FLAVOR										

	0.5	1	1.5	2	2.5	3	3.5	4	4.5	5
SWEET										
ACIDIC										
SPICY										
CITRUS										
CHOCOLATE										
CARAMEL										
BITTER										
SAVORY										

BREW METHOD

DRIP ☐   ESPRESSO ☐   PRESS ☐

POUR-OVER ☐   SIPHON ☐   OTHER _____

NOTES _____
_____
_____
_____
_____
_____
_____
_____
_____
_____

RECOMMEND TO _____
_____
_____
_____
_____
_____
_____
_____
_____
_____

COFFEE NAME _____ DATE _____

BEVERAGE _____

PLACE TASTED _____ PRICE _____

COUNTRY / REGION _____

COMPANY _____

TESTING RATING

```
              0.5  1  1.5  2  2.5  3  3.5  4  4.5  5                    0.5  1  1.5  2  2.5  3  3.5  4  4.5  5
APPEARANCE  [                              ]      SWEET       [                              ]
AROMA       [                              ]      ACIDIC      [                              ]
FLAVOR      [                              ]      SPICY       [                              ]
                                                  CITRUS      [                              ]
                                                  CHOCOLATE   [                              ]
## BREW METHOD                                    CARAMEL     [                              ]
                                                  BITTER      [                              ]
DRIP ☐    ESPRESSO ☐    PRESS ☐                   SAVORY      [                              ]

POUR-OVER ☐    SIPHON ☐    OTHER _____
```

NOTES _____   RECOMMEND TO _____

_____ _____
_____ _____
_____ _____
_____ _____
_____ _____
_____ _____
_____ _____
_____ _____
_____ _____
_____ _____

COFFEE NAME _____ DATE _____

BEVERAGE _____

PLACE TASTED _____ PRICE _____

COUNTRY / REGION _____

COMPANY _____

TESTING RATING

	0.5	1	1.5	2	2.5	3	3.5	4	4.5	5
APPEARANCE										
AROMA										
FLAVOR										

	0.5	1	1.5	2	2.5	3	3.5	4	4.5	5
SWEET										
ACIDIC										
SPICY										
CITRUS										
CHOCOLATE										
CARAMEL										
BITTER										
SAVORY										

BREW METHOD

DRIP ☐   ESPRESSO ☐   PRESS ☐

POUR-OVER ☐   SIPHON ☐   OTHER _____

NOTES _____
_____
_____
_____
_____
_____
_____
_____
_____
_____

RECOMMEND TO _____
_____
_____
_____
_____
_____
_____
_____
_____
_____

COFFEE NAME _____ DATE _____

BEVERAGE _____

PLACE TASTED _____ PRICE _____

COUNTRY / REGION _____

COMPANY _____

TESTING RATING

```
              0.5  1  1.5  2  2.5  3  3.5  4  4.5  5
APPEARANCE   [                                      ]
AROMA        [                                      ]
FLAVOR       [                                      ]
```

```
              0.5  1  1.5  2  2.5  3  3.5  4  4.5  5
SWEET        [                                      ]
ACIDIC       [                                      ]
SPICY        [                                      ]
CITRUS       [                                      ]
CHOCOLATE    [                                      ]
CARAMEL      [                                      ]
BITTER       [                                      ]
SAVORY       [                                      ]
```

BREW METHOD

DRIP ☐   ESPRESSO ☐   PRESS ☐

POUR-OVER ☐   SIPHON ☐   OTHER _____

NOTES _____

_____
_____
_____
_____
_____
_____
_____
_____
_____
_____

RECOMMEND TO _____

_____
_____
_____
_____
_____
_____
_____
_____
_____
_____

COFFEE NAME _____ **DATE** _____

BEVERAGE _____

PLACE TASTED _____ **PRICE** _____

COUNTRY / REGION _____

COMPANY _____

TESTING RATING

```
              0.5  1  1.5  2  2.5  3  3.5  4  4.5  5
APPEARANCE   [                                      ]
AROMA        [                                      ]
FLAVOR       [                                      ]
```

```
              0.5  1  1.5  2  2.5  3  3.5  4  4.5  5
SWEET        [                                      ]
ACIDIC       [                                      ]
SPICY        [                                      ]
CITRUS       [                                      ]
CHOCOLATE    [                                      ]
CARAMEL      [                                      ]
BITTER       [                                      ]
SAVORY       [                                      ]
```

BREW METHOD

DRIP ☐   ESPRESSO ☐   PRESS ☐

POUR-OVER ☐   SIPHON ☐   OTHER _____

NOTES _____

_____
_____
_____
_____
_____
_____
_____
_____
_____

RECOMMEND TO _____

_____
_____
_____
_____
_____
_____
_____
_____
_____

COFFEE NAME _____ DATE _____

BEVERAGE _____

PLACE TASTED _____   PRICE _____

COUNTRY / REGION _____

COMPANY _____

TESTING RATING

```
                0.5  1  1.5  2  2.5  3  3.5  4  4.5  5
APPEARANCE     [                                      ]
AROMA          [                                      ]
FLAVOR         [                                      ]
```

```
            0.5  1  1.5  2  2.5  3  3.5  4  4.5  5
SWEET      [                                      ]
ACIDIC     [                                      ]
SPICY      [                                      ]
CITRUS     [                                      ]
CHOCOLATE  [                                      ]
CARAMEL    [                                      ]
BITTER     [                                      ]
SAVORY     [                                      ]
```

BREW METHOD

DRIP ☐   ESPRESSO ☐   PRESS ☐

POUR-OVER ☐   SIPHON ☐   OTHER _____

NOTES _____

_____
_____
_____
_____
_____
_____
_____
_____
_____
_____

RECOMMEND TO _____

_____
_____
_____
_____
_____
_____
_____
_____
_____
_____

COFFEE NAME _____ **DATE** _____

BEVERAGE _____

PLACE TASTED _____   **PRICE** _____

COUNTRY / REGION _____

COMPANY _____

TESTING RATING

	0.5	1	1.5	2	2.5	3	3.5	4	4.5	5
APPEARANCE										
AROMA										
FLAVOR										

	0.5	1	1.5	2	2.5	3	3.5	4	4.5	5
SWEET										
ACIDIC										
SPICY										
CITRUS										
CHOCOLATE										
CARAMEL										
BITTER										
SAVORY										

BREW METHOD

DRIP ☐   ESPRESSO ☐   PRESS ☐

POUR-OVER ☐   SIPHON ☐   OTHER _____

NOTES _____

_____
_____
_____
_____
_____
_____
_____
_____
_____
_____

RECOMMEND TO _____

_____
_____
_____
_____
_____
_____
_____
_____
_____
_____

COFFEE NAME _____ DATE _____

BEVERAGE _____

PLACE TASTED _____ PRICE _____

COUNTRY / REGION _____

COMPANY _____

TESTING RATING

	0.5 1 1.5 2 2.5 3 3.5 4 4.5 5
APPEARANCE	☐☐☐☐☐☐☐☐☐☐
AROMA	☐☐☐☐☐☐☐☐☐☐
FLAVOR	☐☐☐☐☐☐☐☐☐☐

	0.5 1 1.5 2 2.5 3 3.5 4 4.5 5
SWEET	☐☐☐☐☐☐☐☐☐☐
ACIDIC	☐☐☐☐☐☐☐☐☐☐
SPICY	☐☐☐☐☐☐☐☐☐☐
CITRUS	☐☐☐☐☐☐☐☐☐☐
CHOCOLATE	☐☐☐☐☐☐☐☐☐☐
CARAMEL	☐☐☐☐☐☐☐☐☐☐
BITTER	☐☐☐☐☐☐☐☐☐☐
SAVORY	☐☐☐☐☐☐☐☐☐☐

BREW METHOD

DRIP ☐   ESPRESSO ☐   PRESS ☐

POUR-OVER ☐   SIPHON ☐   OTHER _____

NOTES _____

_____
_____
_____
_____
_____
_____
_____
_____
_____
_____

RECOMMEND TO _____

_____
_____
_____
_____
_____
_____
_____
_____
_____
_____

COFFEE NAME _____ **DATE** _____

BEVERAGE _____

PLACE TASTED _____ **PRICE** _____

COUNTRY / REGION _____

COMPANY _____

TESTING RATING

	0.5	1	1.5	2	2.5	3	3.5	4	4.5	5
APPEARANCE										
AROMA										
FLAVOR										

	0.5	1	1.5	2	2.5	3	3.5	4	4.5	5
SWEET										
ACIDIC										
SPICY										
CITRUS										
CHOCOLATE										
CARAMEL										
BITTER										
SAVORY										

BREW METHOD

DRIP ☐   ESPRESSO ☐   PRESS ☐

POUR-OVER ☐   SIPHON ☐   OTHER _____

NOTES _____

_____
_____
_____
_____
_____
_____
_____
_____
_____
_____

RECOMMEND TO _____

_____
_____
_____
_____
_____
_____
_____
_____
_____
_____

COFFEE NAME _____ DATE _____

BEVERAGE _____

PLACE TASTED _____ PRICE _____

COUNTRY / REGION _____

COMPANY _____

TESTING RATING

	0.5 1 1.5 2 2.5 3 3.5 4 4.5 5
APPEARANCE	▭▭▭▭▭▭▭▭▭▭
AROMA	▭▭▭▭▭▭▭▭▭▭
FLAVOR	▭▭▭▭▭▭▭▭▭▭

	0.5 1 1.5 2 2.5 3 3.5 4 4.5 5
SWEET	▭▭▭▭▭▭▭▭▭▭
ACIDIC	▭▭▭▭▭▭▭▭▭▭
SPICY	▭▭▭▭▭▭▭▭▭▭
CITRUS	▭▭▭▭▭▭▭▭▭▭
CHOCOLATE	▭▭▭▭▭▭▭▭▭▭
CARAMEL	▭▭▭▭▭▭▭▭▭▭
BITTER	▭▭▭▭▭▭▭▭▭▭
SAVORY	▭▭▭▭▭▭▭▭▭▭

BREW METHOD

DRIP ☐   ESPRESSO ☐   PRESS ☐

POUR-OVER ☐   SIPHON ☐   OTHER _____

NOTES

_____
_____
_____
_____
_____
_____
_____
_____
_____
_____

RECOMMEND TO

_____
_____
_____
_____
_____
_____
_____
_____
_____
_____

COFFEE NAME _____ **DATE** _____

BEVERAGE _____

PLACE TASTED _____ **PRICE** _____

COUNTRY / REGION _____

COMPANY _____

TESTING RATING

	0.5	1	1.5	2	2.5	3	3.5	4	4.5	5
APPEARANCE										
AROMA										
FLAVOR										

	0.5	1	1.5	2	2.5	3	3.5	4	4.5	5
SWEET										
ACIDIC										
SPICY										
CITRUS										
CHOCOLATE										
CARAMEL										
BITTER										
SAVORY										

BREW METHOD

DRIP ☐   ESPRESSO ☐   PRESS ☐

POUR-OVER ☐   SIPHON ☐   OTHER _____

NOTES _____

_____
_____
_____
_____
_____
_____
_____
_____
_____
_____

RECOMMEND TO _____

_____
_____
_____
_____
_____
_____
_____
_____
_____
_____

COFFEE NAME _____ DATE _____

BEVERAGE _____

PLACE TASTED _____ PRICE _____

COUNTRY / REGION _____

COMPANY _____

TESTING RATING

	0.5	1	1.5	2	2.5	3	3.5	4	4.5	5
APPEARANCE										
AROMA										
FLAVOR										

	0.5	1	1.5	2	2.5	3	3.5	4	4.5	5
SWEET										
ACIDIC										
SPICY										
CITRUS										
CHOCOLATE										
CARAMEL										
BITTER										
SAVORY										

BREW METHOD

DRIP ☐   ESPRESSO ☐   PRESS ☐

POUR-OVER ☐   SIPHON ☐   OTHER _____

NOTES _____

_____
_____
_____
_____
_____
_____
_____
_____
_____
_____

RECOMMEND TO _____

_____
_____
_____
_____
_____
_____
_____
_____
_____
_____

COFFEE NAME _____   **DATE** _____

BEVERAGE _____

PLACE TASTED _____   **PRICE** _____

COUNTRY / REGION _____

COMPANY _____

TESTING RATING

	0.5	1	1.5	2	2.5	3	3.5	4	4.5	5
APPEARANCE										
AROMA										
FLAVOR										

	0.5	1	1.5	2	2.5	3	3.5	4	4.5	5
SWEET										
ACIDIC										
SPICY										
CITRUS										
CHOCOLATE										
CARAMEL										
BITTER										
SAVORY										

BREW METHOD

DRIP ☐   ESPRESSO ☐   PRESS ☐

POUR-OVER ☐   SIPHON ☐   OTHER _____

NOTES _____

_____

_____

_____

_____

_____

_____

_____

_____

_____

_____

RECOMMEND TO _____

_____

_____

_____

_____

_____

_____

_____

_____

_____

_____

COFFEE NAME _____ DATE _____

BEVERAGE _____

PLACE TASTED _____ PRICE _____

COUNTRY / REGION _____

COMPANY _____

TESTING RATING

```
              0.5  1  1.5  2  2.5  3  3.5  4  4.5  5
APPEARANCE   [                                      ]
AROMA        [                                      ]
FLAVOR       [                                      ]
```

```
              0.5  1  1.5  2  2.5  3  3.5  4  4.5  5
SWEET        [                                      ]
ACIDIC       [                                      ]
SPICY        [                                      ]
CITRUS       [                                      ]
CHOCOLATE    [                                      ]
CARAMEL      [                                      ]
BITTER       [                                      ]
SAVORY       [                                      ]
```

BREW METHOD

DRIP ☐   ESPRESSO ☐   PRESS ☐

POUR-OVER ☐   SIPHON ☐   OTHER _____

NOTES _____

_____
_____
_____
_____
_____
_____
_____
_____
_____
_____

RECOMMEND TO _____

_____
_____
_____
_____
_____
_____
_____
_____
_____
_____

COFFEE NAME _____ DATE _____

BEVERAGE _____

PLACE TASTED _____ PRICE _____

COUNTRY / REGION _____

COMPANY _____

TESTING RATING

	0.5	1	1.5	2	2.5	3	3.5	4	4.5	5
APPEARANCE										
AROMA										
FLAVOR										

	0.5	1	1.5	2	2.5	3	3.5	4	4.5	5
SWEET										
ACIDIC										
SPICY										
CITRUS										
CHOCOLATE										
CARAMEL										
BITTER										
SAVORY										

BREW METHOD

DRIP ☐   ESPRESSO ☐   PRESS ☐

POUR-OVER ☐   SIPHON ☐   OTHER _____

NOTES _____

RECOMMEND TO _____

COFFEE NAME _____ DATE _____

BEVERAGE _____

PLACE TASTED _____ PRICE _____

COUNTRY / REGION _____

COMPANY _____

TESTING RATING

	0.5 1 1.5 2 2.5 3 3.5 4 4.5 5
APPEARANCE	
AROMA	
FLAVOR	

	0.5 1 1.5 2 2.5 3 3.5 4 4.5 5
SWEET	
ACIDIC	
SPICY	
CITRUS	
CHOCOLATE	
CARAMEL	
BITTER	
SAVORY	

BREW METHOD

DRIP ☐   ESPRESSO ☐   PRESS ☐

POUR-OVER ☐   SIPHON ☐   OTHER _____

NOTES _____

RECOMMEND TO _____

COFFEE NAME _____   DATE _____

BEVERAGE _____

PLACE TASTED _____   PRICE _____

COUNTRY / REGION _____

COMPANY _____

TESTING RATING

	0.5	1	1.5	2	2.5	3	3.5	4	4.5	5
APPEARANCE										
AROMA										
FLAVOR										

	0.5	1	1.5	2	2.5	3	3.5	4	4.5	5
SWEET										
ACIDIC										
SPICY										
CITRUS										
CHOCOLATE										
CARAMEL										
BITTER										
SAVORY										

BREW METHOD

DRIP ☐   ESPRESSO ☐   PRESS ☐

POUR-OVER ☐   SIPHON ☐   OTHER _____

NOTES _____   RECOMMEND TO _____

COFFEE NAME _____ DATE _____

BEVERAGE _____

PLACE TASTED _____ PRICE _____

COUNTRY / REGION _____

COMPANY _____

TESTING RATING

	0.5	1	1.5	2	2.5	3	3.5	4	4.5	5
APPEARANCE										
AROMA										
FLAVOR										

	0.5	1	1.5	2	2.5	3	3.5	4	4.5	5
SWEET										
ACIDIC										
SPICY										
CITRUS										
CHOCOLATE										
CARAMEL										
BITTER										
SAVORY										

BREW METHOD

DRIP ☐   ESPRESSO ☐   PRESS ☐

POUR-OVER ☐   SIPHON ☐   OTHER _____

NOTES _____

RECOMMEND TO _____

COFFEE NAME _____ DATE _____

BEVERAGE _____

PLACE TASTED _____   PRICE _____

COUNTRY / REGION _____

COMPANY _____

TESTING RATING

	0.5	1	1.5	2	2.5	3	3.5	4	4.5	5
APPEARANCE										
AROMA										
FLAVOR										

	0.5	1	1.5	2	2.5	3	3.5	4	4.5	5
SWEET										
ACIDIC										
SPICY										
CITRUS										
CHOCOLATE										
CARAMEL										
BITTER										
SAVORY										

BREW METHOD

DRIP ☐   ESPRESSO ☐   PRESS ☐

POUR-OVER ☐   SIPHON ☐   OTHER _____

NOTES _____

RECOMMEND TO _____

COFFEE NAME _____   DATE _____

BEVERAGE _____

PLACE TASTED _____   PRICE _____

COUNTRY / REGION _____

COMPANY _____

TESTING RATING

```
              0.5  1  1.5  2  2.5  3  3.5  4  4.5  5
APPEARANCE   [                                      ]
AROMA        [                                      ]
FLAVOR       [                                      ]
```

BREW METHOD

DRIP ☐   ESPRESSO ☐   PRESS ☐

POUR-OVER ☐   SIPHON ☐   OTHER _____

```
            0.5  1  1.5  2  2.5  3  3.5  4  4.5  5
SWEET      [                                      ]
ACIDIC     [                                      ]
SPICY      [                                      ]
CITRUS     [                                      ]
CHOCOLATE  [                                      ]
CARAMEL    [                                      ]
BITTER     [                                      ]
SAVORY     [                                      ]
```

NOTES _____

_____
_____
_____
_____
_____
_____
_____
_____
_____
_____

RECOMMEND TO _____

_____
_____
_____
_____
_____
_____
_____
_____
_____
_____

COFFEE NAME _____ DATE _____

BEVERAGE _____

PLACE TASTED _____ PRICE _____

COUNTRY / REGION _____

COMPANY _____

TESTING RATING

	0.5	1	1.5	2	2.5	3	3.5	4	4.5	5
APPEARANCE										
AROMA										
FLAVOR										

	0.5	1	1.5	2	2.5	3	3.5	4	4.5	5
SWEET										
ACIDIC										
SPICY										
CITRUS										
CHOCOLATE										
CARAMEL										
BITTER										
SAVORY										

BREW METHOD

DRIP ☐   ESPRESSO ☐   PRESS ☐

POUR-OVER ☐   SIPHON ☐   OTHER _____

NOTES _____

_____

_____

_____

_____

_____

_____

_____

_____

RECOMMEND TO _____

_____

_____

_____

_____

_____

_____

_____

_____

COFFEE NAME _____ **DATE** _____

BEVERAGE _____

PLACE TASTED _____ **PRICE** _____

COUNTRY / REGION _____

COMPANY _____

TESTING RATING

```
              0.5  1  1.5  2  2.5  3  3.5  4  4.5  5
APPEARANCE   [                                      ]
AROMA        [                                      ]
FLAVOR       [                                      ]
```

```
              0.5  1  1.5  2  2.5  3  3.5  4  4.5  5
SWEET        [                                      ]
ACIDIC       [                                      ]
SPICY        [                                      ]
CITRUS       [                                      ]
CHOCOLATE    [                                      ]
CARAMEL      [                                      ]
BITTER       [                                      ]
SAVORY       [                                      ]
```

BREW METHOD

DRIP ☐   ESPRESSO ☐   PRESS ☐

POUR-OVER ☐   SIPHON ☐   OTHER _____

NOTES _____

_____
_____
_____
_____
_____
_____
_____
_____
_____
_____

RECOMMEND TO _____

_____
_____
_____
_____
_____
_____
_____
_____
_____
_____

COFFEE NAME _____   DATE _____

BEVERAGE _____

PLACE TASTED _____   PRICE _____

COUNTRY / REGION _____

COMPANY _____

TESTING RATING

	0.5	1	1.5	2	2.5	3	3.5	4	4.5	5
APPEARANCE										
AROMA										
FLAVOR										

	0.5	1	1.5	2	2.5	3	3.5	4	4.5	5
SWEET										
ACIDIC										
SPICY										
CITRUS										
CHOCOLATE										
CARAMEL										
BITTER										
SAVORY										

BREW METHOD

DRIP ☐   ESPRESSO ☐   PRESS ☐

POUR-OVER ☐   SIPHON ☐   OTHER _____

NOTES _____
_____
_____
_____
_____
_____
_____
_____
_____
_____
_____
_____

RECOMMEND TO _____
_____
_____
_____
_____
_____
_____
_____
_____
_____
_____
_____

COFFEE NAME _____ DATE _____

BEVERAGE _____

PLACE TASTED _____ PRICE _____

COUNTRY / REGION _____

COMPANY _____

TESTING RATING

```
              0.5  1  1.5  2  2.5  3  3.5  4  4.5  5
APPEARANCE  [                                        ]
AROMA       [                                        ]
FLAVOR      [                                        ]
```

```
            0.5  1  1.5  2  2.5  3  3.5  4  4.5  5
SWEET     [                                        ]
ACIDIC    [                                        ]
SPICY     [                                        ]
CITRUS    [                                        ]
CHOCOLATE [                                        ]
CARAMEL   [                                        ]
BITTER    [                                        ]
SAVORY    [                                        ]
```

BREW METHOD

DRIP ☐   ESPRESSO ☐   PRESS ☐

POUR-OVER ☐   SIPHON ☐   OTHER _____

NOTES _____

_____
_____
_____
_____
_____
_____
_____
_____
_____

RECOMMEND TO _____

_____
_____
_____
_____
_____
_____
_____
_____
_____

COFFEE NAME _____ DATE _____

BEVERAGE _____

PLACE TASTED _____   PRICE _____

COUNTRY / REGION _____

COMPANY _____

TESTING RATING

```
            0.5 1 1.5 2 2.5 3 3.5 4 4.5 5
APPEARANCE [                              ]
AROMA      [                              ]
FLAVOR     [                              ]
```

```
            0.5 1 1.5 2 2.5 3 3.5 4 4.5 5
SWEET      [                              ]
ACIDIC     [                              ]
SPICY      [                              ]
CITRUS     [                              ]
CHOCOLATE  [                              ]
CARAMEL    [                              ]
BITTER     [                              ]
SAVORY     [                              ]
```

BREW METHOD

DRIP ☐   ESPRESSO ☐   PRESS ☐

POUR-OVER ☐   SIPHON ☐   OTHER _____

NOTES _____

_____
_____
_____
_____
_____
_____
_____
_____
_____
_____

RECOMMEND TO _____

_____
_____
_____
_____
_____
_____
_____
_____
_____
_____

COFFEE NAME _____ DATE _____

BEVERAGE _____

PLACE TASTED _____ PRICE _____

COUNTRY / REGION _____

COMPANY _____

TESTING RATING

```
              0.5  1  1.5  2  2.5  3  3.5  4  4.5  5                    0.5  1  1.5  2  2.5  3  3.5  4  4.5  5
APPEARANCE  [                                    ]   SWEET      [                                    ]
AROMA       [                                    ]   ACIDIC     [                                    ]
FLAVOR      [                                    ]   SPICY      [                                    ]
                                                     CITRUS     [                                    ]
                                                     CHOCOLATE  [                                    ]
                                                     CARAMEL    [                                    ]
                                                     BITTER     [                                    ]
                                                     SAVORY     [                                    ]
```

BREW METHOD

DRIP ☐   ESPRESSO ☐   PRESS ☐

POUR-OVER ☐   SIPHON ☐   OTHER _____

NOTES _____

RECOMMEND TO _____

COFFEE NAME _____ DATE _____

BEVERAGE _____

PLACE TASTED _____ PRICE _____

COUNTRY / REGION _____

COMPANY _____

TESTING RATING

	0.5	1	1.5	2	2.5	3	3.5	4	4.5	5
APPEARANCE										
AROMA										
FLAVOR										

	0.5	1	1.5	2	2.5	3	3.5	4	4.5	5
SWEET										
ACIDIC										
SPICY										
CITRUS										
CHOCOLATE										
CARAMEL										
BITTER										
SAVORY										

BREW METHOD

DRIP ☐   ESPRESSO ☐   PRESS ☐

POUR-OVER ☐   SIPHON ☐   OTHER _____

NOTES _____

_____
_____
_____
_____
_____
_____
_____
_____
_____
_____
_____

RECOMMEND TO _____

_____
_____
_____
_____
_____
_____
_____
_____
_____
_____
_____

COFFEE NAME _____ DATE _____

BEVERAGE _____

PLACE TASTED _____ PRICE _____

COUNTRY / REGION _____

COMPANY _____

TESTING RATING

	0.5 1 1.5 2 2.5 3 3.5 4 4.5 5
APPEARANCE	▭▭▭▭▭▭▭▭▭▭
AROMA	▭▭▭▭▭▭▭▭▭▭
FLAVOR	▭▭▭▭▭▭▭▭▭▭

	0.5 1 1.5 2 2.5 3 3.5 4 4.5 5
SWEET	▭▭▭▭▭▭▭▭▭▭
ACIDIC	▭▭▭▭▭▭▭▭▭▭
SPICY	▭▭▭▭▭▭▭▭▭▭
CITRUS	▭▭▭▭▭▭▭▭▭▭
CHOCOLATE	▭▭▭▭▭▭▭▭▭▭
CARAMEL	▭▭▭▭▭▭▭▭▭▭
BITTER	▭▭▭▭▭▭▭▭▭▭
SAVORY	▭▭▭▭▭▭▭▭▭▭

BREW METHOD

DRIP ☐   ESPRESSO ☐   PRESS ☐

POUR-OVER ☐   SIPHON ☐   OTHER _____

NOTES _____

RECOMMEND TO _____

COFFEE NAME _____   DATE _____

BEVERAGE _____

PLACE TASTED _____   PRICE _____

COUNTRY / REGION _____

COMPANY _____

TESTING RATING

```
              0.5  1  1.5  2  2.5  3  3.5  4  4.5  5
APPEARANCE  [                                      ]
AROMA       [                                      ]
FLAVOR      [                                      ]
```

```
            0.5  1  1.5  2  2.5  3  3.5  4  4.5  5
SWEET     [                                      ]
ACIDIC    [                                      ]
SPICY     [                                      ]
CITRUS    [                                      ]
CHOCOLATE [                                      ]
CARAMEL   [                                      ]
BITTER    [                                      ]
SAVORY    [                                      ]
```

BREW METHOD

DRIP ☐   ESPRESSO ☐   PRESS ☐

POUR-OVER ☐   SIPHON ☐   OTHER _____

NOTES _____
_____
_____
_____
_____
_____
_____
_____
_____
_____
_____

RECOMMEND TO _____
_____
_____
_____
_____
_____
_____
_____
_____
_____
_____

COFFEE NAME _____ **DATE** _____

BEVERAGE _____

PLACE TASTED _____ **PRICE** _____

COUNTRY / REGION _____

COMPANY _____

TESTING RATING

	0.5	1	1.5	2	2.5	3	3.5	4	4.5	5
APPEARANCE										
AROMA										
FLAVOR										

	0.5	1	1.5	2	2.5	3	3.5	4	4.5	5
SWEET										
ACIDIC										
SPICY										
CITRUS										
CHOCOLATE										
CARAMEL										
BITTER										
SAVORY										

BREW METHOD

DRIP ☐   ESPRESSO ☐   PRESS ☐

POUR-OVER ☐   SIPHON ☐   OTHER _____

NOTES _____

_____
_____
_____
_____
_____
_____
_____
_____
_____

RECOMMEND TO _____

_____
_____
_____
_____
_____
_____
_____
_____
_____

COFFEE NAME _____ DATE _____

BEVERAGE _____

PLACE TASTED _____ PRICE _____

COUNTRY / REGION _____

COMPANY _____

TESTING RATING

	0.5	1	1.5	2	2.5	3	3.5	4	4.5	5
APPEARANCE										
AROMA										
FLAVOR										

BREW METHOD

DRIP ☐   ESPRESSO ☐   PRESS ☐

POUR-OVER ☐   SIPHON ☐   OTHER _____

	0.5	1	1.5	2	2.5	3	3.5	4	4.5	5
SWEET										
ACIDIC										
SPICY										
CITRUS										
CHOCOLATE										
CARAMEL										
BITTER										
SAVORY										

NOTES _____

_____
_____
_____
_____
_____
_____
_____
_____
_____
_____

RECOMMEND TO _____

_____
_____
_____
_____
_____
_____
_____
_____
_____
_____

COFFEE NAME _____ DATE _____

BEVERAGE _____

PLACE TASTED _____ PRICE _____

COUNTRY / REGION _____

COMPANY _____

TESTING RATING

	0.5	1	1.5	2	2.5	3	3.5	4	4.5	5
APPEARANCE										
AROMA										
FLAVOR										

	0.5	1	1.5	2	2.5	3	3.5	4	4.5	5
SWEET										
ACIDIC										
SPICY										
CITRUS										
CHOCOLATE										
CARAMEL										
BITTER										
SAVORY										

BREW METHOD

DRIP ☐   ESPRESSO ☐   PRESS ☐

POUR-OVER ☐   SIPHON ☐   OTHER _____

NOTES _____

RECOMMEND TO _____

COFFEE NAME _____ DATE _____

BEVERAGE _____

PLACE TASTED _____ PRICE _____

COUNTRY / REGION _____

COMPANY _____

TESTING RATING

	0.5	1	1.5	2	2.5	3	3.5	4	4.5	5
APPEARANCE										
AROMA										
FLAVOR										

	0.5	1	1.5	2	2.5	3	3.5	4	4.5	5
SWEET										
ACIDIC										
SPICY										
CITRUS										
CHOCOLATE										
CARAMEL										
BITTER										
SAVORY										

BREW METHOD

DRIP ☐   ESPRESSO ☐   PRESS ☐

POUR-OVER ☐   SIPHON ☐   OTHER _____

NOTES _____
_____
_____
_____
_____
_____
_____
_____
_____
_____
_____

RECOMMEND TO _____
_____
_____
_____
_____
_____
_____
_____
_____
_____
_____

COFFEE NAME _____ **DATE** _____

BEVERAGE _____

PLACE TASTED _____ **PRICE** _____

COUNTRY / REGION _____

COMPANY _____

TESTING RATING

	0.5	1	1.5	2	2.5	3	3.5	4	4.5	5
APPEARANCE										
AROMA										
FLAVOR										

	0.5	1	1.5	2	2.5	3	3.5	4	4.5	5
SWEET										
ACIDIC										
SPICY										
CITRUS										
CHOCOLATE										
CARAMEL										
BITTER										
SAVORY										

BREW METHOD

DRIP ☐   ESPRESSO ☐   PRESS ☐

POUR-OVER ☐   SIPHON ☐   OTHER _____

NOTES _____

_____
_____
_____
_____
_____
_____
_____
_____

RECOMMEND TO _____

_____
_____
_____
_____
_____
_____
_____
_____

COFFEE NAME _____   DATE _____

BEVERAGE _____

PLACE TASTED _____   PRICE _____

COUNTRY / REGION _____

COMPANY _____

TESTING RATING

```
              0.5  1  1.5  2  2.5  3  3.5  4  4.5  5
APPEARANCE  [                                        ]
AROMA       [                                        ]
FLAVOR      [                                        ]
```

BREW METHOD

DRIP ☐   ESPRESSO ☐   PRESS ☐

POUR-OVER ☐   SIPHON ☐   OTHER _____

```
          0.5  1  1.5  2  2.5  3  3.5  4  4.5  5
SWEET     [                                        ]
ACIDIC    [                                        ]
SPICY     [                                        ]
CITRUS    [                                        ]
CHOCOLATE [                                        ]
CARAMEL   [                                        ]
BITTER    [                                        ]
SAVORY    [                                        ]
```

NOTES _____

_____
_____
_____
_____
_____
_____
_____
_____
_____
_____

RECOMMEND TO _____

_____
_____
_____
_____
_____
_____
_____
_____
_____
_____

COFFEE NAME _____   DATE _____

BEVERAGE _____

PLACE TASTED _____   PRICE _____

COUNTRY / REGION _____

COMPANY _____

TESTING RATING

```
              0.5  1  1.5  2  2.5  3  3.5  4  4.5  5
APPEARANCE   [                                      ]
AROMA        [                                      ]
FLAVOR       [                                      ]
```

```
           0.5  1  1.5  2  2.5  3  3.5  4  4.5  5
SWEET     [                                      ]
ACIDIC    [                                      ]
SPICY     [                                      ]
CITRUS    [                                      ]
CHOCOLATE [                                      ]
CARAMEL   [                                      ]
BITTER    [                                      ]
SAVORY    [                                      ]
```

BREW METHOD

DRIP ☐   ESPRESSO ☐   PRESS ☐

POUR-OVER ☐   SIPHON ☐   OTHER _____

NOTES
_____
_____
_____
_____
_____
_____
_____
_____
_____
_____

RECOMMEND TO
_____
_____
_____
_____
_____
_____
_____
_____
_____
_____

COFFEE NAME _____ **DATE** _____

BEVERAGE _____

PLACE TASTED _____ **PRICE** _____

COUNTRY / REGION _____

COMPANY _____

TESTING RATING

```
              0.5  1  1.5  2  2.5  3  3.5  4  4.5  5
APPEARANCE   [                                      ]
AROMA        [                                      ]
FLAVOR       [                                      ]
```

BREW METHOD

DRIP ☐   ESPRESSO ☐   PRESS ☐

POUR-OVER ☐   SIPHON ☐   OTHER _____

```
            0.5  1  1.5  2  2.5  3  3.5  4  4.5  5
SWEET      [                                      ]
ACIDIC     [                                      ]
SPICY      [                                      ]
CITRUS     [                                      ]
CHOCOLATE  [                                      ]
CARAMEL    [                                      ]
BITTER     [                                      ]
SAVORY     [                                      ]
```

NOTES _____

_____
_____
_____
_____
_____
_____
_____
_____
_____

RECOMMEND TO _____

_____
_____
_____
_____
_____
_____
_____
_____
_____

COFFEE NAME _____ DATE _____

BEVERAGE _____

PLACE TASTED _____ PRICE _____

COUNTRY / REGION _____

COMPANY _____

TESTING RATING

	0.5 1 1.5 2 2.5 3 3.5 4 4.5 5
APPEARANCE	▢▢▢▢▢▢▢▢▢▢
AROMA	▢▢▢▢▢▢▢▢▢▢
FLAVOR	▢▢▢▢▢▢▢▢▢▢

	0.5 1 1.5 2 2.5 3 3.5 4 4.5 5
SWEET	▢▢▢▢▢▢▢▢▢▢
ACIDIC	▢▢▢▢▢▢▢▢▢▢
SPICY	▢▢▢▢▢▢▢▢▢▢
CITRUS	▢▢▢▢▢▢▢▢▢▢
CHOCOLATE	▢▢▢▢▢▢▢▢▢▢
CARAMEL	▢▢▢▢▢▢▢▢▢▢
BITTER	▢▢▢▢▢▢▢▢▢▢
SAVORY	▢▢▢▢▢▢▢▢▢▢

BREW METHOD

DRIP ☐   ESPRESSO ☐   PRESS ☐

POUR-OVER ☐   SIPHON ☐   OTHER _____

NOTES _____

RECOMMEND TO _____

COFFEE NAME _____   **DATE** _____

BEVERAGE _____

PLACE TASTED _____   **PRICE** _____

COUNTRY / REGION _____

COMPANY _____

TESTING RATING

	0.5	1	1.5	2	2.5	3	3.5	4	4.5	5
APPEARANCE										
AROMA										
FLAVOR										

BREW METHOD

DRIP ☐   ESPRESSO ☐   PRESS ☐

POUR-OVER ☐   SIPHON ☐   OTHER _____

	0.5	1	1.5	2	2.5	3	3.5	4	4.5	5
SWEET										
ACIDIC										
SPICY										
CITRUS										
CHOCOLATE										
CARAMEL										
BITTER										
SAVORY										

NOTES _____

_____
_____
_____
_____
_____
_____
_____
_____
_____
_____

RECOMMEND TO _____

_____
_____
_____
_____
_____
_____
_____
_____
_____
_____

COFFEE NAME _____ DATE _____

BEVERAGE _____

PLACE TASTED _____ PRICE _____

COUNTRY / REGION _____

COMPANY _____

TESTING RATING

```
              0.5  1  1.5  2  2.5  3  3.5  4  4.5  5
APPEARANCE  [                                        ]
AROMA       [                                        ]
FLAVOR      [                                        ]
```

```
          0.5  1  1.5  2  2.5  3  3.5  4  4.5  5
SWEET     [                                        ]
ACIDIC    [                                        ]
SPICY     [                                        ]
CITRUS    [                                        ]
CHOCOLATE [                                        ]
CARAMEL   [                                        ]
BITTER    [                                        ]
SAVORY    [                                        ]
```

BREW METHOD

DRIP ☐   ESPRESSO ☐   PRESS ☐

POUR-OVER ☐   SIPHON ☐   OTHER _____

NOTES _____

RECOMMEND TO _____

COFFEE NAME _____ DATE _____

BEVERAGE _____

PLACE TASTED _____ PRICE _____

COUNTRY / REGION _____

COMPANY _____

TESTING RATING

	0.5	1	1.5	2	2.5	3	3.5	4	4.5	5
APPEARANCE										
AROMA										
FLAVOR										

	0.5	1	1.5	2	2.5	3	3.5	4	4.5	5
SWEET										
ACIDIC										
SPICY										
CITRUS										
CHOCOLATE										
CARAMEL										
BITTER										
SAVORY										

BREW METHOD

DRIP ☐   ESPRESSO ☐   PRESS ☐

POUR-OVER ☐   SIPHON ☐   OTHER _____

NOTES

_____
_____
_____
_____
_____
_____
_____
_____
_____
_____

RECOMMEND TO

_____
_____
_____
_____
_____
_____
_____
_____
_____
_____

COFFEE NAME _____   DATE _____

BEVERAGE _____

PLACE TASTED _____   PRICE _____

COUNTRY / REGION _____

COMPANY _____

TESTING RATING

```
                0.5  1  1.5  2  2.5  3  3.5  4  4.5  5
APPEARANCE  [                                         ]
AROMA       [                                         ]
FLAVOR      [                                         ]
```

BREW METHOD

DRIP ☐   ESPRESSO ☐   PRESS ☐

POUR-OVER ☐   SIPHON ☐   OTHER _____

```
            0.5  1  1.5  2  2.5  3  3.5  4  4.5  5
SWEET     [                                         ]
ACIDIC    [                                         ]
SPICY     [                                         ]
CITRUS    [                                         ]
CHOCOLATE [                                         ]
CARAMEL   [                                         ]
BITTER    [                                         ]
SAVORY    [                                         ]
```

NOTES _____   RECOMMEND TO _____

_____   _____
_____   _____
_____   _____
_____   _____
_____   _____
_____   _____
_____   _____
_____   _____
_____   _____
_____   _____

COFFEE NAME _____   DATE _____

BEVERAGE _____

PLACE TASTED _____   PRICE _____

COUNTRY / REGION _____

COMPANY _____

TESTING RATING

```
              0.5  1  1.5  2  2.5  3  3.5  4  4.5  5
APPEARANCE   [                                      ]
AROMA        [                                      ]
FLAVOR       [                                      ]
```

```
              0.5  1  1.5  2  2.5  3  3.5  4  4.5  5
SWEET        [                                      ]
ACIDIC       [                                      ]
SPICY        [                                      ]
CITRUS       [                                      ]
CHOCOLATE    [                                      ]
CARAMEL      [                                      ]
BITTER       [                                      ]
SAVORY       [                                      ]
```

BREW METHOD

DRIP ☐   ESPRESSO ☐   PRESS ☐

POUR-OVER ☐   SIPHON ☐   OTHER _____

NOTES _____

_____
_____
_____
_____
_____
_____
_____
_____
_____
_____

RECOMMEND TO _____

_____
_____
_____
_____
_____
_____
_____
_____
_____
_____

COFFEE NAME _____   DATE _____

BEVERAGE _____

PLACE TASTED _____   PRICE _____

COUNTRY / REGION _____

COMPANY _____

TESTING RATING

```
              0.5  1  1.5  2  2.5  3  3.5  4  4.5  5
APPEARANCE   [                                      ]
AROMA        [                                      ]
FLAVOR       [                                      ]
```

```
              0.5  1  1.5  2  2.5  3  3.5  4  4.5  5
SWEET        [                                      ]
ACIDIC       [                                      ]
SPICY        [                                      ]
CITRUS       [                                      ]
CHOCOLATE    [                                      ]
CARAMEL      [                                      ]
BITTER       [                                      ]
SAVORY       [                                      ]
```

BREW METHOD

DRIP ☐   ESPRESSO ☐   PRESS ☐

POUR-OVER ☐   SIPHON ☐   OTHER _____

NOTES _____

_____
_____
_____
_____
_____
_____
_____
_____
_____
_____

RECOMMEND TO _____

_____
_____
_____
_____
_____
_____
_____
_____
_____
_____

COFFEE NAME _____ DATE _____

BEVERAGE _____

PLACE TASTED _____   PRICE _____

COUNTRY / REGION _____

COMPANY _____

TESTING RATING

	0.5	1	1.5	2	2.5	3	3.5	4	4.5	5
APPEARANCE										
AROMA										
FLAVOR										

	0.5	1	1.5	2	2.5	3	3.5	4	4.5	5
SWEET										
ACIDIC										
SPICY										
CITRUS										
CHOCOLATE										
CARAMEL										
BITTER										
SAVORY										

BREW METHOD

DRIP ☐   ESPRESSO ☐   PRESS ☐

POUR-OVER ☐   SIPHON ☐   OTHER _____

NOTES _____
_____
_____
_____
_____
_____
_____
_____
_____
_____
_____

RECOMMEND TO _____
_____
_____
_____
_____
_____
_____
_____
_____
_____
_____

COFFEE NAME _____ **DATE** _____

BEVERAGE _____

PLACE TASTED _____ **PRICE** _____

COUNTRY / REGION _____

COMPANY _____

TESTING RATING

	0.5	1	1.5	2	2.5	3	3.5	4	4.5	5
APPEARANCE										
AROMA										
FLAVOR										

	0.5	1	1.5	2	2.5	3	3.5	4	4.5	5
SWEET										
ACIDIC										
SPICY										
CITRUS										
CHOCOLATE										
CARAMEL										
BITTER										
SAVORY										

BREW METHOD

DRIP ☐   ESPRESSO ☐   PRESS ☐

POUR-OVER ☐   SIPHON ☐   OTHER _____

NOTES _____

_____
_____
_____
_____
_____
_____
_____
_____
_____

RECOMMEND TO _____

_____
_____
_____
_____
_____
_____
_____
_____
_____

COFFEE NAME _____   **DATE** _____

BEVERAGE _____

PLACE TASTED _____   **PRICE** _____

COUNTRY / REGION _____

COMPANY _____

TESTING RATING

```
                0.5  1  1.5  2  2.5  3  3.5  4  4.5  5
APPEARANCE  [                                         ]
AROMA       [                                         ]
FLAVOR      [                                         ]
```

```
              0.5  1  1.5  2  2.5  3  3.5  4  4.5  5
SWEET     [                                         ]
ACIDIC    [                                         ]
SPICY     [                                         ]
CITRUS    [                                         ]
CHOCOLATE [                                         ]
CARAMEL   [                                         ]
BITTER    [                                         ]
SAVORY    [                                         ]
```

BREW METHOD

DRIP ☐   ESPRESSO ☐   PRESS ☐

POUR-OVER ☐   SIPHON ☐   OTHER _____

NOTES _____

_____

_____

_____

_____

_____

_____

_____

_____

_____

_____

_____

RECOMMEND TO _____

_____

_____

_____

_____

_____

_____

_____

_____

_____

_____

_____

COFFEE NAME _____ DATE _____

BEVERAGE _____

PLACE TASTED _____ PRICE _____

COUNTRY / REGION _____

COMPANY _____

TESTING RATING

	0.5	1	1.5	2	2.5	3	3.5	4	4.5	5
APPEARANCE										
AROMA										
FLAVOR										

	0.5	1	1.5	2	2.5	3	3.5	4	4.5	5
SWEET										
ACIDIC										
SPICY										
CITRUS										
CHOCOLATE										
CARAMEL										
BITTER										
SAVORY										

BREW METHOD

DRIP ☐   ESPRESSO ☐   PRESS ☐

POUR-OVER ☐   SIPHON ☐   OTHER _____

NOTES _____

_____
_____
_____
_____
_____
_____
_____
_____
_____
_____

RECOMMEND TO _____

_____
_____
_____
_____
_____
_____
_____
_____
_____
_____

COFFEE NAME _____ DATE _____

BEVERAGE _____

PLACE TASTED _____ PRICE _____

COUNTRY / REGION _____

COMPANY _____

TESTING RATING

```
              0.5  1  1.5  2  2.5  3  3.5  4  4.5  5
APPEARANCE  [                                        ]
AROMA       [                                        ]
FLAVOR      [                                        ]
```

```
            0.5  1  1.5  2  2.5  3  3.5  4  4.5  5
SWEET     [                                        ]
ACIDIC    [                                        ]
SPICY     [                                        ]
CITRUS    [                                        ]
CHOCOLATE [                                        ]
CARAMEL   [                                        ]
BITTER    [                                        ]
SAVORY    [                                        ]
```

BREW METHOD

DRIP ☐   ESPRESSO ☐   PRESS ☐

POUR-OVER ☐   SIPHON ☐   OTHER _____

NOTES _____
_____
_____
_____
_____
_____
_____
_____
_____
_____
_____

RECOMMEND TO _____
_____
_____
_____
_____
_____
_____
_____
_____
_____
_____